# PSIONIC MEDICINE

# PSIONIC MEDICINE

The study and treatment of the causative factors in illness

J.H. REYNER BSc, DIC, FIEE
in collaboration with
GEORGE LAURENCE MRCS, LRCP,
FRCS (Edin) FIPsiMed
and CARL UPTON LDS (Birm), FIPsiMed

Revised by
KEITH SOUTER MB, ChB, FRCGP, MIPsiMed,
MHMA, Dip Med Ac

INDEX COMPILED BY ANN GRIFFITHS

SAFFRON WALDEN
THE C.W. DANIEL COMPANY LIMITED

First published in Great Britain in 2001
by The C.W. Daniel Company Limited
1 Church Path, Saffron Walden,
Essex, CB10 1JP, United Kingdom

© The Psionic Medical Society 2001

ISBN  0 85207 342 9

The authors have asserted their rights under the Copyright Design
and Patent Act 1988 (and under any comparable provision of any
comparable law in any jurisdiction whatsoever) to be identified as
the author of this work.

So far as may legally effectively be provided no liability of any kind
or nature whatsoever, whether in negligence, under statute, or
otherwise, is accepted by the authors or the publishers for the
accuracy or safety of any of the information or advice contained in,
or in any way relating to any part of the content, of this book.

All rights reserved.  No part of this publication may be reproduced,
stored in a retrieval system, or transmitted in any form or by any
means, electronic, mechanical, photocopying, recording, or
otherwise, without the prior permission of the copyright holder.

The Random House Group Limited supports The Forest Stewardship
Council (FSC®), the leading international forest certification organisation.
Our books carrying the FSC label are printed on FSC® certified paper.
FSC is the only forest certification scheme endorsed by the leading
environmental organisations, including Greenpeace. Our
paper procurement policy can be found at
www.randomhouse.co.uk/environment

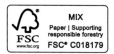

Printed and bound in Great Britain by Clays Ltd, St Ives PLC
Production in association with
Book Production Consultants plc, 25–27 High Street,
Chesterton, Cambridge CB4 1ND.
Typeset by Cambridge Photosetting Services

# Contents

# Acknowledgements

There are many people who contribute to the making of a book. I would like to thank J.H. Reyner, George Laurence and Carl Upton, for giving us the first book. Thanks to Dr Gordon Flint, the President of the Institute of Psionic Medicine, for his preface, Dr Farley Spink, the Dean of the Institute of Psionic Medicine for his chapter on Miasms and Toxins, Mr Mark Elliott, the first veterinary psionic practitioner, for his chapter on Psionic Veterinary Practice.

Appreciation goes to Dr Pam Tatham, current Secretary of the Institute of Psionic Medicine, and to Dr Geoffrey Goodyear, immediate past Secretary, for their comments on the manuscript. Also thanks to fellow members, Dr Carol Brierly, Mr David Hooper, Dr Vincent Mainey, Dr Peter Mansfield, Dr Leon Wyman and Dr David Williams for the insights they have given in their lectures and writings. Thanks also to Dr Anne Wynne-Simmons, a long-time associate and supporter of Psionic Medicine.

The support of the Psionic Medical Society is much appreciated. In particular, thanks to Sir Charles Jessel, President of the Society for his unstinting enthusiasm, support and leadership. Thanks also to Dr Solveig McIntosh, Vice-President of the Society, Mr John Fryer, Secretary of the Society, and Mr Edwin Barclay, Treasurer of the Society. Thanks in no small measure to the members of the Psionic Medical Society for their interest and support of the method.

Special thanks to my friend and colleague, Quincy Day Rabôt, for our many useful and enjoyable chats about energy medicine and Traditional Chinese Medicine.

A huge thank you to Professor Ervin Laszlo, Patron of the Psionic Medical Society, for so eloquently describing his vision of the new science, which is so eruditely formulated in his Psi-Field Hypothesis, which forms the second chapter of this book.

Thank you to our publishers, The C.W. Daniel Co Ltd, who as always make book producing seem such an effortless art.

And finally, thank you to Mollie, Rachel, Kate, Ruth and Andrew, respectively, mother, wife and children for putting up with yet another book project.

K.S.

# Foreword by Professor Ervin Laszlo

It is a genuine pleasure to write a Foreword to a book that makes a rare and significant contribution to our individual and collective well-being. *Psionic Medicine: the study and treatment of causative factors in illness* acquaints the reader with the nature and accomplishments of that uniquely advanced branch of the science of healing that goes under the name of Psionic Medicine.

I have the privilege of first-hand knowledge of the efficacy of this form of medicine, having been under psionic medical care for nearly a decade. My personal experience confirms an insight I had also reached independently, by way of inference from the latest findings of the physical and biological sciences. It is that the living organism is not a mere mechanism, nor merely a biochemical system, but a complex system of molecular, cellular and field components. This is relevant, for Psionic Medicine acts not on the molecular or cellular components of the organism, but on the field that governs its molecular and cellular processes.

The affirmation of a field as a basic element in the living organism is not new in the history of twentieth century biology. As early as 1925, Viennese biologist. Paul Weiss, inspired by Wolfgang Koehler's Gestalt theory, applied the field concept to processes of limb regeneration in amphibians, and later he generalised the concept to all forms of ontogenesis. On the basis of his experimental work Weiss concluded that the emergence of organs and tissues during development indicates that the emerging parts assume patterned spatial relations exhibited in geometric features of position, proportion, and orientation. These, he said, are 'field actions'. Each species has its own morphogenetic field, and each individual's morphogenetic field is a nested hierarchy of subsidiary fields.

Likewise in the 1920s Russian biologist, Alexander Gurwitch, noted that the role of individual cells in embryogenesis is determined neither by their own properties nor by their relations to neighbouring cells, but by a factor that seems to involve the entire developmental system. This, he said, is a system-wide force field created by the mutual effect of the individual force fields associated with cells. The boundaries of the field of an embryo, for example, do not coincide with the boundaries of the embryo itself: they penetrate beyond it. Embryogenesis, Gurwitch said, occurs within the embryo's morphogenetic field.

In 1934 Conrad Waddington introduced the idea of 'individuation fields' active in the formation of organs, and in 1957 extended the field idea to 'chreods', the developmental pathways of embryogenesis. This notion was elaborated by René Thom in mathematical models that represent the state toward which the organism is developing by 'basins of attraction' within morphogenetic fields. In the 1950s Harold Saxton Burr of Yale University measured the electromagnetic properties of what he called the L (life) field, and his co-workers showed that this field vanishes at the death of the organism.

Although biological field theories were pioneered in the 1920s and attained wide popularity in mid century, the physical properties of the fields were not well-defined and in subsequent decades interest in them declined. In embryology, for example, biochemical methods did not enable researchers to discover the nature of the fields that would govern limb polarity, neural patterning, lens induction, and other developmental processes. Field concepts came to be regarded as speculative, and in recent years only a handful of investigators persisted in producing biological field theories. For the most part, biologists shifted their attention to the biochemistry of specific genetic mechanisms, a powerful approach that yielded a plethora of practical applications.

In the last few decades, however, though less known than research into genetic codes and mechanisms, field concepts resurfaced at the leading edge of biological research. Canadian biologist, Brian Goodwin, advanced a field-based concept of regeneration and reproduction, processes in which a whole is generated from a part. These, he said, cannot be viewed solely in terms of germ plasm and DNA, but must be seen as arising from the field properties of living organisms. Biological fields generate spatial orders that influence the activity of genes, and gene activity in turn influences the fields. The field is the unit of form and organisation, while the molecules and cells that make up the body are the units of composition: fields structure them into the order that characterises the organism. Life is a 'sacred dance' of cells within organisms, and of organisms within their milieu, where biological fields keep the partners in step. Rupert Sheldrake, in turn, put forward the 'hypothesis of formative causation' according to which morphic fields are associated with all living organisms and are responsible for their ongoing morphogenesis.

Of course, the presence of complex fields associated with cellular matter has never been contested in biology — the evidence uncovered in biophysics brooks no contradiction. However, in the mainstream of the biological sciences, the role and function of the electric, magnetic, and other fields associated with cellular matter have not been considered of major relevance for the functioning of the organism, merely secondary effects produced by biochemically communicating cells, tissues, and organs. The current rediscovery of biological fields constitutes a fundamental shift in emphasis. It is like the 'figure-ground switch' described by Gestalt psychologists, where the visual perception of an image is snapped back and forth between seeing one of its aspects as figure and another as ground. In mainstream biology and medicine the figure is the assembly of organic molecules constituting the cell, while the fields produced by cellular communication — insofar as they are taken into account at all — are seen as the real but physiologically and medically insignificant background. By contrast, in leading-edge research, the same as in alternative medicine, the figure is the field, and the molecules, cells and organs on which it acts, the ground.

The current Gestalt-switch comes about both in view of the experimental discovery of wide-ranging and quasi-instant interaction within the organism, and in light of alternative medicine's discovery of subtle yet effective interaction between doctor and patient. It appears that the living organism is an instantaneously interconnected system that maintains itself in its milieu as a whole, suffers damage as a whole, but can also heal itself as a whole. These features depend crucially on the field coordination of the organism's vast number and wide variety of molecular and cellular processes.

Recognising the primacy of fields in the maintenance and reestablishment of health is fundamental for contemporary medicine. In this concept the functioning of the organism does not approximate the workings of a machine, hence simple kinetic manipulations have corrective value only in specific cases such as, for example, those treated by chiropractors. The functioning of the organism is also not fully and adequately represented by the concept of a biochemical system, and consequently the allopathic treatments prescribed by conventional Western medicine likewise have limited application. The complement to mechanistic and biochemical treatment is alternative medicine's field-based therapy, convincingly exemplified in psionic medicine.

Psionic medicine's motto *'tolle causam'* (Search for the Cause) is eminently warranted. Treating the field of the organism means treating the basic aspect of the living state, the one that in the cybernetic sense 'governs' the orchestrated interaction of the organism's myriad biochemical components. Sickness is an impairment of the integrity of the organism's governing field, and it is properly and effectively treated as such. By comparison, treating the biochemical processes of the patient means treating the entailed consequences of the impairment of his or her biofield, rather than the cause of the ailment, which is the impairment of the field itself. Conventional treatment, illustrated for instance by the use of broad-spectrum antibiotics, involves unnecessarily drastic measures, like shooting at mosquitos with cannon-balls. Treating the organism's governing field is far less invasive and is more efficient.

A further aspect of psionic medicine which merits comment is its functioning across any hitherto tested finite distances. This, at first sight, mind-boggling, remote-diagnostic — and in some cases also remote-healing — feature is accounted for when we recognise that the field embedding and governing the cellular and multicellular organism is a quantum field. This is not an ad hoc assumption: it follows from the finding that the scope of biological coherence transcends the scope of biochemical signal transmission, even if some biochemical signalling is remarkably effective. The coherence exhibited by living organisms (the simultaneous and quasi-instant correlation of all its parts with all its other parts) is a form of quantum-coherence — the kind of coherence that can only be explained in reference to the concepts and laws of quantum theory. Biologists in the emerging discipline of quantum biology speak of the 'macroscopic wavefunction of the organism' and view living tissue as a Bose-Einstein condensate where effects analogous to superfluidity and superconductivity occur at ordinary temperatures.

Theories and concepts coming to the fore at cutting-edge biology indicate that the organism's biofield is a specific manifestation of a more fundamental quantum field — a field that mediates interaction throughout physical nature. The biofield is a local structure within a wider and more basic field: the field that, independently of each other, both this writer and the founders of Psionic Medicine termed 'psi-field'. The writer's theory of the psi field offers a natural science account of the space- and time-transcending transmission of information coming to light in the practice of psionic medicine.

Psionic Medicine heralds the dawn of a new era in medical practice, with health-maintaining and curative potentials that are a significant addition to the repertory of treatment developed in biochemical medicine. In Psionic Medicine the critical factor is not chemistry and surgical intervention — though such methods remain indicated in some cases — but subtle 'informational' inputs that affect the patient's biofield. The book in the hands of the reader provides a remarkably clear and concise overview of what psionic medicine is, how it works, and why it deserves the kind of attention that presently only molecular and genetics-based breakthroughs are accorded. It merits serious and urgent attention by the general lay public and the medical profession alike.

November 2000

# Preface to the Third Edition

## By Gordon Flint, BSc, MB, ChB, D(Obst),RCOG, FIPsiMed

I feel very privileged and honoured to have been invited to write this preface to Dr Keith Souter's skilful revision of the two previous editions of *Psionic Medicine*.

One of the most important words in this new book is 'interconnectedness' and the reader can only enjoy being led through the history of medicine from ancient times representing Eastern philosophy, via Hippocrates and more Western culture, to this twenty-first century and the energy medicine into which we are committing ourselves, aided by the researches of Professor Ervin Laszlo in his Psi-Field Hypothesis.

Each aspirant to successful psionic practice brings to it his or her own current expertise, via the training we have received in the medical, dental and veterinary sciences, backed by years of clinical experience, first in orthodox then, later, in homoeopathic study and later still in the techniques of psionic practice, with perhaps further experience in other branches of science and areas such as acupuncture and medical hypnosis.

The first and all-important skill must be in the use of our dowsing sense, which, like the basic five, we possess at the moment of birth — yet, while it will take the first few years of our life to acquire a good measure of skill in interpreting our immediate environment through sight, hearing, smell, taste and touch, it may be a few decades before we can make any practical use of our ability to dowse — and as can be seen from a standard distribution chart, about 10 per cent will be naturals with very considerable ability, 10 per cent may well achieve nothing of note, while the rest of us, with practice, can improve to very acceptable levels as this sense becomes every bit as reliable as the basic five.

I had the privilege of being trained by Carl Upton and I once said to him, 'I wish I had known about Psionic Medicine ten years ago.' His instant response was, 'Gordon, ten years ago, you weren't ready for this.' And of course, he was absolutely right.

Where Homocopathy is concerned, a good knowledge and experience of the basic philosophy, principles and practice, as introduced and taught by Samuel Hahnemann, is essential and time must be spent attending courses of instruction, whenever possible, at various teaching centres around the country. Nevertheless, none of the three big names in Psionic Medicine — Laurence, Upton or Westlake had specific qualifications in this subject and Dr Farley Spink, our current Dean, was the first amongst us to introduce his particular talent for and experience in classical homoeopathy, to the great advantage of us all.

Mark Elliott, our first Veterinary practitioner, has made a very special contribution to our overall knowledge of psionic practice and who knows what the content of some future edition of this book may be.

At the moment, we believe that when revalidation and reaccreditation are on the minds of all of us, it is right to restrict training in the psionic method to doctors, dentists and veterinary practitioners — but, in the foreseeable future, in these days when there is so much talk about genetically modified (some would say mutilated) crops, may it be that we will need to seek help from other sources, and Botany and Crop Farming come to mind. J.E.R. McDonagh, whose ideas and work so stimulated our Founder President, George Laurence, insisted that the most important starting point was the soil and good healthy soil, possessing a good healthy microbiological 'climate'. Such soil would virtually guarantee healthy crops, leading to healthy stock and of course the potential for healthy people. Needless to say, this also includes clean, drinkable water, uncontaminated by potentially poisonous residues or additives.

Initial training in Psionic Medicine will last for at least a year, while experience is gained. Thereafter, continuing practice produces a quite enormous degree of job satisfaction as the various challenges produced by patients in their quite unique and individual ways encourage us to determine, like Laurence, WHY people are ill.

# Preface to the Second Edition

### By Carl Upton, LDS (Birm), FIPsiMed

Alexis Carrel, formerly of the Rockefeller Institute for Medical Research, in his book, *Man, the Unknown*, writes that there are two kinds of health: natural and artificial. Scientific medicine, he says, has given to man artificial health, and protection against most infectious diseases. It is a marvellous gift. Yet man should not need to rely on continual medication with its special diets and synthetic chemicals. If body and mind are in harmony the organism functions in a naturally healthy manner. There are indeed certain individuals who appear to possess a natural immunity, which not only resists infection but delays the onset of senescence. We have to discover their secret.

George Laurence would have endorsed this view wholeheartedly. Conventional medicine is apt to consider the body as a rather fallible machine of which the component parts are liable to breakdown, necessitating frequent repair or even replacement. Laurence, however, regarded it as a highly intelligent structure enlivened by an appropriate but invisible pattern of vital force; but from a variety of causes, some inherited, some acquired by accident or misuse, this underlying pattern can become distorted, resulting in a departure from the natural state of health.

His great achievement was the discovery of a means of communicating with this unseen pattern and the development of the technique which he called Psionic Medicine, whereby derangements of the vital force can be detected and possibly corrected. He was able by simple and direct analysis to prescribe suitable homoeopathic remedies, which he found acted in a harmonious and non-toxic way and which were capable of removing the often deeply entrenched subtle causes of disease. He pursued this inspired course almost to the end of his long life. He died on 11th October 1978, shortly after his ninety-eighth birthday.

It is clearly desirable that doctors who recognise the truth of those ideas should be able to be trained in the basic techniques of the psionic medical approach, so that they can begin to apply the methods in practice. In fact this is now happening at the Institute of Psionic Medicine, though not without problems. Apart from the difficulty of accepting any departure from established habit, some sacrifice of time and money will be required while learning the necessary skills. Yet, despite this, there is growing interest on the part of both doctors and the public, and many thousands of patients have been successfully treated.

Psionic Medicine is natural medicine, requiring both the use of the intuitive senses and the manifold provision of nature in the remedies it provides. It is not a 'fringe' medicine, but a uniquely practical method of using these natural facilities to identify and treat the hidden causes of the diseases that plague mankind today.

# Preface to the First Edition

*By George Laurence MRCP, LRCP, FRCS (Edin), FIPsiMed*

I find it most gratifying that a scientist of Mr Reyner's standing should be so deeply convinced of the value of psionic methods of diagnosis.

As a doctor for over 65 years, I am disappointed with the lack of progress in medicine, especially as compared with the advances in surgery and other allied fields. Every day countless treatments and cures are advertised, but the majority of these are based on new synthetic chemicals — and causation has been ignored. The psionic principle looks for the cause of deviation from normal health before trying to deal with symptoms.

It is my hope that the book will stimulate interest in this important branch of medical science.

# PART ONE

# THE SCIENCE
# AND PHILOSOPHY OF
# PSIONIC MEDICINE

# A New Dimension
## in Medicine

*'Nature abhors a vacuum.'*

**François Rabelais (c.1494—1553)**

There are epochs in medical history when the trend of knowledge is significantly changed. One can cite Harvey's classical treatise on the circulation of the blood in 1628, or the microbiological studies of Louis Pasteur and the discovery of the X-ray by Wilhelm Röntgen in the nineteenth century. The twentieth century then saw the discovery of penicillin by Fleming in 1928, the breaking of the DNA code by Watson and Crick in 1953, and the first heart transplant by Dr Christiaan Barnard in 1967. At the beginning of the twenty-first century scientists are working towards the decipherment of the human genome.

Concurrently, there has been a vast expansion of knowledge of the physical structure of living matter, both in respect of the intricate structure of the cells and the communication between them, as a result of which medical practice has been able to devise new treatments for many bodily ailments, often with spectacular success. These very successes, however, have tended to create an undue reliance on the material aspects of medicine, in the belief that a full understanding of the physical mechanisms will ultimately provide a cure for all the ailments of the flesh. Indeed, molecular biology and genetic engineering are advancing so rapidly that it is estimated that within a few decades we should hold the key to the genetic basis for many cancers and chronic diseases.

This is an illusion for, although an intelligent application of material knowledge can produce an amelioration of the conditions, the clinical symptoms are really only the physical evidence of some disturbance of the vital energy of the body. This is not in itself a new philosophy, having been held, if not always acknowledged, for at least 2,500 years. In fact, Hippocrates, revered as the Father of Medicine, is reported to have said that disease does not appear purely as a malady (*pathos*), but is significantly accompanied by an exertion (*ponos*) by the body itself to restore the disturbed equilibrium of its functions. This inherent healing power is known as *Vis Medicatrix Naturae*, and the enlightened physician is well aware that his true role is merely to assist it, by creating the correct circumstances for it to operate in as unimpeded a fashion as is possible.

One should be quite clear about this: it is the individual's own healing mechanisms that truly deal with the illness, not the surgeon's, physician's or whatever health professional is involved. A surgeon may remove a tumour, but the body heals the wounds. Similarly, a physician may give a drug, but it is the patient's body that responds to it.

These healing mechanisms, referred to in physiology as the body's 'homoeostatic', or self-regulatory mechanisms, are always operating in order to do their best for the individual. They regulate such things as metabolism, temperature, fluid and mineral balance, blood chemistry, and the overall production and disposal of body cells. When the body is stressed in some way, then they automatically attempt to restore some sort of balance. Very often the individual is able to perceive these changes as being out of the ordinary, or unpleasant. These are the symptoms of illness as the body attempts to correct the problem. The trouble is that the mechanisms rarely return completely back to normal. Although function is restored to 'near-normal service' it is often at a cost. That cost may be in a reduction of function, alteration of function or alteration in structure. Essentially, in the majority of cases, rather than a rebalancing, it is a compensation that takes place.

Western orthodox medicine is firmly based on a reductionist model. Clearly, this has been successful in many fields of endeavour, but it does have undoubted limitations. It rejects the concept of a *'vital principle'*, instead considering the body to be a complex integration of cells, tissues, organs and systems, united by biochemical control and overseen by an internal biological computer, the brain. In many other successful medical systems (and globally, Western orthodox medicine and surgery only come fourth as suppliers of medical care), the vital principle is pretty well central to their philosophy. An increasing number of doctors, and an even greater number of patients, believe that this limitation is positively harmful to the development of medicine.

## Biochemical or biophysical control

On purely logical grounds, the limitations of a biochemical-dominated model are only too clear. The human body is composed of an incredibly large number of cells, working in different ways, living for different times, according to the tissue type that they belong to. Every schoolchild knows the old chestnut about the body being replaced every seven years. This means that over a seven-year period all of the soft tissue cells of the body will have been replaced at least once. Effectively, at any one time there is a significant amount of growth, repair, reproduction and elimination of dying cells going on throughout one's body. A biochemical control of this complexity, to maintain a fine balance to keep the cellular integrity of the whole system intact, is beyond belief.

No, while the chemical controls that we know about undoubtedly go a long way towards explaining how the cells of the body can be integrated, we have to postulate another more encompassing control. Some form of energetic information system, or energy field, perhaps.

We mentioned above that a *vital principle* is central to many systems of medicine. The Chinese know it as *Chi* and the Indian yogis as *Prana*. In addition, it has been postulated or 'rediscovered' by various individuals throughout history. For example, Paracelsus called it *Munia*, the alchemists termed it *Vital Fluid* and Baron Von Reichenbach, the German chemist who discovered creosote, called it *Odyle*. In the twentieth century Wilhelm Reich called it *Orgone*, Rudolph Steiner termed it the *Etheric Formative Force*, and yet others labelled it *Bioplasma*, *Biological Plasma* or *Bio-Field*.

In all of these cases, although there is a slightly different interpretation, it is regarded as a form of energy which permeates living creatures during life and which is an integral part of their whole being. It is thought to be a field within and around the organism, which produces a sort of *Etheric Body*.

Such an energy 'body' seems to function as an information system, operating as a template for foetal development, subsequent growth and development, tissue organisation and for trouble-shooting tissue repair.

## The pyramid of medicine

Since medicine is a practice as old as mankind itself, it is appropriate to use a model in keeping both with its antiquity and its development — the pyramid.

If you read any book about the history of medicine you will see that the foundation of scientific medicine was laid when man first began to understand anatomical structure, through dissection and a study of *Anatomy*. Observation and experimentation then led to deductions about the function of the organs and their anatomical structures. This gave rise to the science of *Physiology*. With ever-increasing sophistication in instrumentation and applied chemical knowledge, the science of *Biochemistry* developed. The role of the mind has always been a vexing question in its relationship to the body, but with the development of the new science of Mind-Body Medicine or *Psychoneuroimmunology* (PNI),[1] we begin to see how thought processes may influence neurological, hormonal and immunological function. These four sciences then form what has been perceived as the pyramid of medicine. The widespread belief is that this edifice of knowledge, which is thought to be complete to the best of man's ability, would explain all about the body and the body's needs. The biochemical reactions in the cells would explain how they worked to account for the body's physiological functioning of the anatomical structures. And of course, the mind could exert its effects through the PNI routes.

However, as we have implied earlier, this is more of a *mastaba*[2] than a pyramid (Figure 1). Yet still, like the mastabas of ancient Egypt, it has served its function up to a point. It was necessary first to construct these structures in order to understand and later plan how to complete the full structure.

It seems entirely appropriate at this point to introduce the great Imhotep (c. 2,800BC), high priest of Ra, Royal Architect, Personal Physician and Grand Vizier to the Pharaoh Djozer of the Third Dynasty. Sir William Osler, the doyen of twentieth-century physicians wrote that he was: 'the first figure of a physician to stand out clearly from the mists of antiquity.' In later centuries he was deified as a god of healing and was identified by the Greeks with their god Aesculapius. To have attained deification he had undoubtedly raised the practice of medicine in some substantial way. And indeed, as the architect of Pharaoh Djoser's pyramid, he symbolically enhanced Egypt's kudos for millennia. He redesigned the mastaba of Djoser to create the famous Step Pyramid at Saqqara, thereby giving the world the pyramid as an icon of ancient wisdom.

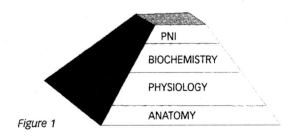

*Figure 1*

And so, one can see that the *bioenergetic model* is a logical extension of the biochemical model of orthodox medicine, analogous to the development of the mastaba into a pyramid. The traditional sciences take us so far, but they leave us tantalisingly short of proper understanding. Effectively, we need to add a capstone to achieve our pyramid. That capstone is the organising energy, or bioenergy, and its appropriate science should be what for now we shall call energy medicine (Figure 2).

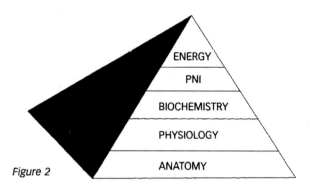

Figure 2

## The energy field

Regeneration, the manner in which organisms reproduce parts that are damaged or lost, was one of the areas that intrigued biologists and proved a fascinating field of research in the early twentieth century. In 1907 the zoologist, H.V. Wilson, performed the ultimate experiment in regeneration, when he forced a small sponge through a fine sieve, thus separating the cells and destroying the intercellular organisation of the organism. After separation, however, the isolated cells wandered around until they came together again in an unorganised aggregation, which within a few weeks reformed itself into a sponge of the original kind.

In the 1920s, Alexander Gurwitch postulated the existence of a form-generating or *morphogenetic* field, which was involved in the embryological development of organisms. It was his concept that this organising field, a sort of developmental blueprint, determined the role of particular cells during embryogenesis, rather than the individual properties of the cells themselves.

Over the following decades various workers researched this concept of a *biofield*, which would be capable of regulating the growth and development of cells and issues within organisms. Notable among these was the Yale biologist, Dr Harold Saxton Burr, who over a period of 40 years conducted numerous experiments on organisms, ranging from simple slime moulds to man himself. Burr concluded that this biofield, which he termed the *L-field* (Life-field), was the basic blueprint of all life, and that every organism had one, which both organised and directed the total structure of the organism.

Using highly sophisticated electronic apparatus Burr demonstrated that the L-field could be measured and mapped out. Not only that, but his researches on humans showed that physical and mental conditions were mirrored by changes in the L-field measurements.

Interestingly in 1950, using an 'electro-metric test' based upon Burr's work, Dr Louis Langman of the Department of Obstetrics and Gynaecology at New York University published a study to see whether measuring the field forces in women could have any diagnostic value in detecting cancers. He and his team concluded that such testing was in fact highly accurate, simple to perform and worthy of further study and research.

Yet another of his collaborators, Leonard Ravitz, claimed that the L-field disappeared just before physical death, the conclusion being that when the organisational life force disappeared, life could not be sustained.

In the 1960s biophysicists, led by Viktor Inyushin at Alma-Ata in the former Soviet Union, performed extensive investigations on what they called the 'energy-body'. One of the stimuli towards this research had been the discovery of the so-called 'Kirlian effect', which had been discovered by Semyon Kirlian in 1939. Effectively, this was an electrographic process, which produced photographs of the body's aura. They found that the state of the aura varied according to the state of health of the individual.

Inyushin concluded that the energy-body had a physical basis, and that it was an elementary plasma-like constellation made of ionised particles, which he termed *Biological Plasma* or *Bioplasma*. This would, he stated in a formulation of the *Bioplasma Theory*, constitute the ultimate substrate of both chemical and electronic processes, as well as act as a carrier of all the information within the system. And, in explanation of the Kirlian Effect, he felt that because Bioplasma exists in living systems it would be bound to be luminescent in certain circumstances, such as when a strong-pulsed, high-frequency field was applied to the system, as in Kirlian photography.

In the 1980s biologist Rupert Sheldrake proposed his groundbreaking theory of *Morphic Fields*. From the Greek 'morphe' meaning 'form', his concept is of a field of form, pattern, order and structure. These fields he believes organise not only living entities, but also the form of crystals, and of molecules. Thus each type of molecule, be it a protein, such as haemoglobin, or a complex inorganic crystal, has a morphic field of its own. More than that, each organism, each kind of instinct or behaviour, has a field. Thus these morphic fields are perceived as the organising fields of nature. Even what Jung called the collective unconscious could be accommodated into morphic-field theory.

Sheldrake was stimulated to develop his theory because of the many puzzling phenomena in nature that pure chemistry and genes cannot account for. For example, although a single cell contains all the genetic information necessary to multiply into a complete organism, be that a human or a tree, why is the ultimate form always the same?

He was also intrigued by behavioural phenomena, whereby colonies of organisms separated geographically and without contact seemed to develop similar behaviours. This has been demonstrated in birds, apes and humans. For example, after a colony of apes on an island were taught how to wash their food before eating, other colonies with no physical contact or means of communication began to do the same.

This, Sheldrake believes, occurs because of *morphic resonance*, a phenomenon wherein previous structures or the experience of organisms within a species influence contemporary or subsequent similar structures or organisms. Through this resonance, pattern and formative information or influence is transferred across space and time. Thus, living members of a species are linked with former members of the same species and, because the phenomenon of resonance is increased by repetition, an activity or behaviour learned, which was discovered or laboriously learned by earlier individuals, will be quickly learned by others.

Morphic Field theory accounts for this because of two principles, which are integral processes of such fields. Firstly creativity, and secondly habit. Take the bicycle and cycling, for example. Two hundred years ago there was no such thing as a bicycle. Then someone had the concept and the bicycle came into being. This was the creative step. (And how often do we find new 'discoveries' being made independently at almost the same time? We shall return to this point in a moment.) Then people started to learn to ride bicycles. More people learned, probably with great difficulty, but nowadays hundreds of millions of people learn and cycle without giving the process much thought. That is the habit, the repetition within species, which makes the learning process simpler.

Thus, Sheldrake says, nature is essentially habit-forming, and all aspects of nature are based on the principle of habit. One could say, therefore, that the laws of nature are the habits of nature.

## Spontaneous culture links

The student of history cannot help but be amazed at the number of instances when whole cultures have suddenly produced some startling achievement, which has effectively revolutionised their society. And it seems to have happened spontaneously, without any obvious means of connection. Indeed, it seems probable that some of these happenings occurred without one culture having any conception of the existence of the other.

Stone Age artefacts from across the globe indicate, for example, that the first tools, including the first axe, appeared at the same time.

Giant pyramids also appeared across the earth, in Egypt, South America, and Cambodia. Writers such as Graham Hancock put forward a plausible great pan-cultural theory with its roots in a lost civilisation. But, as we shall see, there is another explanation.

Yet it is the development of skills that is so interesting: the cooking of food, cheese-making, bread-making, the production of alcohol, pottery, basket-making, and the general making of similar tools seem to have arisen almost de novo.

And great thinkers. In his book *The Whispering Pond*, Professor Ervin Laszlo describes the great breakthroughs of classical Hebrew, Greek, Chinese and Indian culture, all taking place in a breathtakingly short period of time. The examples are legion: the simultaneous and independent discovery of calculus by both Newton and Leibnitz; the independent formulation of a theory of evolution by Darwin and Wallace; the invention of the telephone by Bell and Gray.

More and more, the theory that we all have access to some sort of 'field' becomes more and more appealing. This is fundamental to our discussion of Psionic Medicine.

## Psionic Medicine

The fundamental aim of Psionic Medicine is encapsulated in the motto of the Psionic Medical Society, *Tolle Causam*, meaning 'Seek the Cause' of the illness. Although the manifestation of the illness is likely to be in the physical, psychological or emotional realm, the cause is often found at the energy level. In other words, it is as if it has become encoded within the energy field, thereby exerting its effect upon the individual by disruption of the organising blueprint of the energy field.

But before considering this further, it would seem appropriate to describe a little about the remarkable doctor who developed this system of medicine that integrates orthodox medicine, homoeopathy and the radiesthetic faculty.

George Laurence qualified from St George's Hospital, London in 1904, having previously studied at Liverpool University. It was while at Liverpool that he was influenced by Sir Oliver Lodge, the Professor of Physics, at the time one of the foremost researchers into the properties of electromagnetic waves. After a series of hospital appointments, in 1915 he passed his Fellowship of the Royal College of Surgeons (Edinburgh), then a year later bought a third share in a practice in Chippenham, Wiltshire. Almost immediately his two senior partners were called up for war service, and he was left to carry on the practice alone, which involved a number of hospital and consultative appointments which continued for nearly 40 years. These included Medical Officer of the Red Cross Hospital and Workhouse, Surgeon of the Cottage Hospital, Medical Superintendent of the Isolation Hospital, Factory Surgeon and Public Vaccinator.

During this time, however, he became increasingly dissatisfied with the orthodox preoccupation with symptoms and drugs. In his own words:

'I had a growing conviction that I did not always know what I was really doing — or rather why I was doing it. In other words, I did not know why people were ill.

'It was fairly easy to treat ordinary infectious diseases and acute ailments, but when it came to chronic disorders such as malignant diseases, rheumatism, degenerate nervous troubles, and other so-called incurable maladies, we did not know the "why", and were reduced to treating names and labels, signs and symptoms, without a clue as to causation; and hence the temporary alleviation of symptoms was the best that I, or any of my contemporaries, could do.'

In his attempts to make sense of the causation of illness, Laurence read widely and felt that the work of three men seemed to offer keys. First was Samuel Hahnemann and his homoeopathic method. Second was Rudolph Steiner, especially in his conception of the formative forces of nature. And third was J.E.R. McDonagh and his Unitary Theory of Disease. (We shall consider their work in fuller detail later.)

At this time, by one of life's chances, he came into contact with Dr Guyon Richards and was introduced to the idea of medical dowsing. This proved to be the key he had been seeking, for he had long been convinced that the physical body is only part of a much larger structure, which is not recognisable by the ordinary senses. He believed that it was within this unmanifest realm that the vital energies operated, and he found that by the use of the pendulum he was able to detect derangements of these energies responsible for the physical and psychological disturbances, which produced the clinical symptoms.

He then found that by an extension of the technique he was able to determine appropriate treatment which would restore the vital harmony — usually, but not necessarily, by homoeopathic medication — and so for the first time was able to formulate a scientific method of diagnosis and treatment of the basic causes of illness. This he developed with patience and assiduity over the years, to develop a system of medicine which has proven to be highly successful over the past 50 years, often disclosing the hidden causes and directing practitioners to the appropriate treatment of many chronic and supposedly incurable diseases.

The system depends essentially on the exercise of the paranormal senses,[3] of which the existence is now scientifically accepted; and, because by convention the Greek letter *psi* had come to be associated in this connotation, Laurence called his system Psionic Medicine.

## Pathology in Psionic Medicine

Psionic Medicine is basically an integrated system, which links orthodox medicine, homoeopathy and radiesthesia, or the dowsing faculty. The main emphasis is on chronic, that is, long standing and persistent, disease.

In order to explain this a little more, let us reconsider our two 'pyramids' of medicine, both the incomplete and the complete form. In orthodox medicine we make a diagnosis, which usually takes account of the effect of the illness on structure, function, biochemical aberration and feeling (respectively, anatomy, physiology, biochemistry and psychology or PNI). Treatment then consists of affecting the main level at which this occurs. If the problem is one of altered structure, then surgery is indicated. If it is of function or biochemical aberration then medical treatment may be necessary. If it is perceived as being psychological, then psychological or psychiatric intervention may be considered. And of course, in cases of conditions affecting all levels, such as in cancer, then all types of intervention may be needed.

Now for many people this approach may be precisely what is required. Their condition may be adequately controlled. For others, however, the condition is never controlled and they live on with a chronic or progressive illness which fails to respond to orthodox interventions.

In Psionic Medicine, the apex of the pyramid of medicine is seen to be the energetic side of the individual, their energy-body or energy field. It is the experience of psionic practitioners that when orthodox treatments fail, they fail because the problem exists and persists in the energetic blueprint, the organising energy field that governs growth, repair and the self-regulating mechanisms of the person. Unless the taints are removed, then the individual may experience ongoing physical, emotional and psychological problems.

Let us consider the most extreme form of physical illness, cancer. Orthodox treatment will possibly comprise surgery to remove the physical tumour and restore physical function, followed by chemotherapy and radiotherapy to kill off any remaining cancer cells. If at some later stage cancer is found to have progressed, it is assumed that the spread is secondary to some remaining cancer tissue which was not removed at operation, or from cancerous cells which were not killed off by the chemotherapy and radiotherapy.

In Psionic Medicine, such a recurrence would not be accounted to a failure of removal of the physical tumour, but to persistence of some pathological *process*, which had not been removed. This process emanates from a taint in the energy field, which would continue to operate to produce a sort of trickle-down effect in the pyramid. Thus, the recurrence is not necessarily a spread, but a continuation of the disease process. In other words it would occur because the cause had neither been found nor treated. Essentially, without knowledge even of the existence of the apex of the pyramid, of the energetic side of the individual, orthodox treatment in chronic disease can rarely be anything other than temporary alleviation.

This simplistic explanation can be seen to occur in all manner of ailments, from cancer to other progressive and degenerative diseases.

Psionic Medicine aims to track down the cause of chronic disease by pinpointing the nature of the pathological aberrations within the energy field of the individual. These aberrations may be inherited from many generations back or acquired throughout the lifetime of the individual.

### What happens in Psionic Medicine?

As mentioned earlier, Psionic Medicine integrates orthodox and homoeopathic medicine with radiesthesia, or the dowsing faculty. To do this, a specimen from the patient, usually hair or blood, is used by the psionic practitioner to tune into the individual's energy psi-field. The basic tools for doing this consist of a pendulum, a measuring chart, a series of diagnostic charts, and a set of pathological and treatment witnesses, or samples in diagnostic phials.

The practitioner uses his or her intuitive faculty, with the pendulum as an indicator, to compare the patient's specimen with that of the pathological specimens. In this way, by mentally asking the right questions, the practitioner can, like a detective, pinpoint the causative factors of the illness. Then, in a similar manner, he can ask appropriate questions leading to the necessary treatment, which is usually homoeopathic (since these are energetic remedies capable of affecting the energetic body) in order to remove the pathological toxin (or toxins), thereby permitting the self-regulating or self-healing mechanisms of the individual to come into operation.

Thus, in terms of our pyramid model, because the taint is removed, the trickle-down effect (the disease process) is halted and the self-regulating or self-healing process should calm feelings, correct biochemical aberration, improve function and, *possibly*, rectify structural impediments.

## Psi in Psionic Medicine

The radiesthetic, or dowsing, faculty is essentially an Altered State of Consciousness (ASC), albeit not a full trance state as one might achieve in hypnosis or meditation. One maintains consciousness in order to formulate appropriate and accurate questions, while 'letting-go' sufficiently in order to receive answers by way of an ideomotor (involuntary) response which results in a pendulum movement.

Three things are worthy of note here. Firstly, in the diagnostic arm of the process one is contacting the patient's psi-field, often at a considerable distance, in order to ascertain what disturbances are present, which ones are relevant, and how they are producing illness. Secondly, the key into the patient's psi-field is their witness of blood or hair. No matter how far apart the witness is from the patient in space or time, there is a connection that reflects the current energetic state of the individual. And thirdly, in the determination of treatment, one is asking questions of an informational system which is infinitely more knowledgeable than the practitioner himself. It is not a case of accessing a memory within the practitioner's own mind or own neurological circuitry.

It seems as if the practitioner tunes into two things during this slightly ASC, the first being the patient's individual psi-field, the second being an infinitely huge information system or field which interconnects practitioner, the patient's sample and the patient, or all of their fields. To achieve this, the tuning-in depends upon a connection between the patient and their witness (or their sample).

As we shall see soon, the concept of an interconnected universe explains much about this fascinating branch of medicine.

## A Theory of Everything or a Grand Unified Theory

When we talk about diagnosis and treatment determination at a distance it is easy to think that we are using a paradigm that has more in keeping with magic than science. This would imply that it is not scientific, which is not the case at all. Indeed, Psionic Medicine can very well claim to be at the cutting edge of science, or indeed, of the New Medicine. Let us now venture into the realms of theoretical physics, for this is highly relevant to our discussion.

Up until the 1990s it was almost universally agreed by theoretical physicists that all matter was made up of atoms and subatomic particles, which were held together by four fundamental forces.

First was the *gravitational force*, which keeps our feet on the earth, stops the sun from exploding and the galaxies from scattering. Second was the *electromagnetic force*, which we harness to power our lights, our homes and our cities. Third was the *weak nuclear force*, which is responsible for radioactive decay. This we use in nuclear medicine, in the use of radioactive tracers in our highly sophisticated diagnostic scanners. Fourth was the *strong nuclear force*, which is demonstrated by the power of the sun, the power within the atom. In the 1990s Sidney Sheldon, Steven Weinberg and Abdus Salam demonstrated that the weak nuclear force and the electromagnetic force were manifestations of a single force, called the *electroweak force*.

The way in which these three fundamental forces operate is of monumental importance in science. But just what is their connection? Indeed, can they all be unified into a single super-force?

There are two main theories, which have each partially explained the nature of these forces. One is the *Quantum Theory* and the other is Einstein's *General Relativity*. They deal with opposite ends of the spectrum, however, because Quantum Theory deals with the realm of the microcosm, the subatomic world, whereas General Relativity explains the macrocosm, the nature of the Big Bang, galaxies and black holes. Quantum Theory explains forces as packets or quanta of energy, whereas General Relativity explains forces as deformations of space-time. Interestingly, you can take either one and derive all of the laws of physics and chemistry from it. You can build the entire scientific edifice from one of the theories — but not from both!

This vexing problem consumed all of Albert Einstein's energy over the last 30 years of his life. He pursued a theory which he never finished, but which he proposed to call the *Unified Field Theory*. Effectively, it was to be a Theory of the Universe. It is a quest that has absorbed the careers of countless theoretical physicists since then.

In the 1970s and 1980s it looked as if a possible solution had presented itself with the development of *Superstring Theory*. The basis of this theory was that all matter is composed of superstrings, which occupy a single point in space-time at any one time. This seemed compatible with both Quantum Theory and General Relativity, except that it could only work if there were 10 dimensions. However, the *Kaluza-Klein Theory* allows for this possibility if the extra dimensions (other than the three spatial ones and the one of time) are curled up into an infinitely small space. It was conjectured that, just before the Big Bang, there was an empty but unstable 10-dimensional universe. This split into two fragments, our known four-dimensional universe and a six-dimensional universe. The universe made the quantum leap to another universe causing the six dimensions to curl up and the four-dimensional universe to expand. This rapid expansion at some point caused the Big Bang. Current thinking is that, rather than this being the creation of everything, it was in fact an aftershock of the collapse of the ten-dimensional universe.

There have been five 'String' theories to date, culminating in the unification of them into a single *M-Theory* in 1994. However, M-Theory only holds true if there were 11 dimensions. Indeed, theoretical physicists are now talking about the possibility of a twelfth dimension.

With these mind-boggling theories (which are of course not testable, because it is impossible to measure dimensions which are smaller than an atom) it would have seemed that a *Grand Unification Theory*, or *Theory of Everything*, had been achieved. Or at least a Theory of Everything about the origins of the universe, the nature of elementary particles and the forces between them. But that is not really even close to a true Theory of Everything, is it?

## The interconnected universe

From the very beginning there were many conflicting interpretations of Quantum Theory. A major paradox was shown by Werner Heisenberg, who was awarded the Nobel Prize in 1943 for his work, which included his formulation of the *Uncertainty principle*. Essentially, this meant that it was not possible at the same time to measure a particle's position as well as its momentum.

Then in 1964 another landmark was reached with the publication of *Bell's Theorem of Interconnectedness*. This created a revolution in thought, because it showed that there are objective, non-local connections in the universe. To put it simply, *if two particles that originated from the same source* interact, they will interact forever (as if their wave functions, having become entangled, remain tangled forever). Thus, two such particles, even separated by a huge distance too far apart for a light signal to travel between them, will still interact, and two measurements can be related instantaneously. There is *non-local* interconnection. Many experiments have now confirmed Bell's theorem.

This is of monumental importance, since all matter comes from the Big Bang, implying that at the quantum level the entire realm of physicality is interconnected.

Professor David Bohm, theoretical physicist and a protégé of

Einstein, wrote widely on this concept of connection and inter-connection. In his book *Wholeness and the Implicate Order*, he pro-posed the concept of 'undivided wholeness' as the true reality. In other words, that the universe is not a collection of separate but coupled parts, and is a complicated web of 'relations' between parts of the unified whole. Essentially he postulates that the uni-verse is constructed on the same principles as a hologram, where the entire information of the universe is contained in each of its parts.

According to Bohm's theory, although phenomena seem to be disconnected and unrelated, this is an illusion of our perception. The true reality is one of 'unity', where all things are linked and are part of the same implicate order, although the connectedness may escape the perception of our senses. Thus, the holographic principle occurs throughout nature,[4] as a feature of the holo-graphic universe.

In his book *The Whispering Pond*, Professor Ervin Laszlo says that 'the basic concept — the veritable kingpin — of genuine uni-fied theories is universal interconnection. Indeed, the very possi-bility of such a theory hinges on finding the field in the universe that would connect atoms and galaxies, mice and men, brains and minds, and feed back information from each to all, and from all to each.'

## The psi-field

There are many paradoxes observed from all of the sciences (physical, biological, psychological and even sociological) that simply cannot be explained unless there is some subtle inter-connection. Only a universal field of some sort, an interconnect-ing field, could explain these paradoxes. But just what could it be and where could it exist?

In our above discussion we have considered current thinking about matter. But we must now also consider that other aspect of reality, namely, space. For countless years it has been thought that space was just that, nothingness, a vacuum. Science has discovered that it is not that at all. It is in fact a *plenum*, which means that it is a filled space, or that it contains something. Scientists now talk about it as the *quantum vacuum*.

Space is filled with an intense energy that is known as the 'zero-point field' (ZPF). Beyond or underlying this, Ervin Laszlo postulates that there is a fundamental field of which the ZPF is a manifestation. This fundamental field is informational in that it has records of everything that has ever happened within it, and it is absolutely interconnecting. It is, therefore, holographic in that any part is interconnected with any other part. It could accurately be termed the *vacuum-based zero-point holofield*.

Laszlo felt that this name would be unduly cumbersome and, since 'it is both a fundamental element in reality and a factor that enters into all our interactions with that reality, it deserves nothing less than a Greek letter.' That letter he chose was $\Psi$, or Psi.

The choice of Psi was not random. In choosing it he admits that it was partly 'because it refers to — and perhaps explains — psi phenomena. This, however, is too easy: the universal holofield does considerably more than convey some varieties of extrasensory information; it also connects quanta and organisms, brains and minds and entire peoples and cultures. The rationale for using $\Psi$ goes beyond parapsychology; it goes beyond psychology and neurophysiology, even biology and ecology. It embraces physics and cosmology, and the full range of the contemporary sciences.'

In Psionic Medicine we routinely tune into the individual's own energy or personal psi-field in order to ascertain the nature of the energy distortions which are affecting them physically, emotionally and psychologically. We do this by means of a specimen which, although remote from the patient, is yet in contiguity, or is interconnected with him via the non-local connections we have been discussing. We also tap into the greater psi-field which Ervin Laszlo has so elegantly described, and which he writes about in the next chapter.

[1]Psychoneuroimmunology (PNI), sometimes also referred to as Psychoneuro-endocrinoimmunology (PNEI) is a developing science linking up mind, brain, hormones and the immune system. Candace Pert, a neuroscientist who discovered the opiate receptor, pioneered research on how the chemicals inside our bodies form a dynamic communication between the mind and the body. As the mouthful of a name suggests, it is a discipline which attracts workers from many fields of study. See Further Reading.

[2]Mastaba – an unfinished, flat-topped bench tomb, the forerunner of the later pyramid design.

[3]Paranormal senses in this context mean simply beyond that of the usually recognised five senses. We shall consider this later in the chapter on Intuition, Extra-Sensory Perception and Psi Phenomena.

[4]*The holographic theory of mind* – a theory founded by Karl Pribram of Stanford Medical School. He began with the ground-breaking work of Karl Lashley, who found that when parts of the brains of animals were removed, there were predictable losses in the functions of vision, appetite, sleep, etc, but no such effect on memory. Pribram conducted many experiments on perception and concluded that when the brain encodes an image it does so in a similar manner to that of a hologram. Further research indicates that other senses such as hearing, smell and touch, may also be processed holographically.

# Psi-Field Hypothesis: A Concise Restatement

## Professor Ervin Laszlo

## 1. Basic considerations

The hypothesis put forward here is based on a holistic concept of the scientifically knowable world. In this concept reality is not fragmentable to fundamentally divergent layers or levels. The observable phenomena are the result of a sequential and occasionally non-linear process of development, linking the basic physical sphere of reality with other, emergent spheres, such as those of life, mind and society. Consequently, all phenomena can be seen to have a physical basis. This, however, does not entail the reduction of phenomena of life and mind to physical processes. The hypothesis requires only that the basic laws and regularities that govern the evolution of the diverse spheres of reality be universal, that is, that they apply to physical, biological, psychological, as well as societal phenomena alike. By this token emergent phenomena are not reduced to their physical origins, merely their interactions are traced to universal (i.e., trans-disciplinary) laws and processes.

### 1.1 INTERCONNECTIONS IN SPACE AND TIME

The empirical realms of physics, the same as those of biology and the human sciences, are not yet fully explored; some findings remain anomalous for the mainstream theories. It appears that the greater part of those anomalies is due to interconnections among phenomena that are not properly accounted for in the currently received conceptions.[1] For example:

In *physics*, it is found that elementary particles in identical quantum states possess non-locality: they are instantly interconnected over finite — and possibly considerable — distances. Photons emitted one by one interfere with one another as simultaneous waves; electrons in superconductors flow in a highly coherent manner taking on identical wave-functions; and electrons are instantly and non-dynamically correlated in the energy shells of atomic nuclei.

In *biology*, it appears that if changes in the environment require major changes in the adaptive plan of the species, those changes are produced on occasion through massive and highly co-ordinated — apparently non-random — genetic mutations. Moreover the morphology, and even the genetic information, of widely different species exhibits striking isomorphies hardly credible in a process of random and disconnected mutation and natural selection within the known time frames.

In the sphere of *mind and consciousness*, current research suggests that the range of human experience exceeds the range traditionally assigned to the sensory organs and the brain. In particular circumstances people appear able to recall any, and perhaps all, of their experiences; and on occasion they seem able to affect each other's mental and bodily states across space and time.

These and related anomalies suggest that phenomena in the physical, the biological, and the psychological realm are subtly but effectively linked. Given such interconnections, we can understand how microparticles can be informed of each other's state within given systems of co-ordinates; how the genome of living organisms can be linked with the relevant aspects of the environment; and how human brains and minds can communicate with one another across space and time.

## 1.2 THE NOTION OF AN INTERCONNECTING FIELD

Some interconnections link parts of elements of one and the same system; others link discrete systems across space and time. If these connections are real rather than illusory, they need to be accounted for by the same type of constructs as other — gravitational, electromagnetic, and nuclear — forms of interaction, that is, by universal exchange forces.[2]

In contemporary physics the universal exchange forces are usually interpreted as classical fields. But the classical fields cannot account for the kind of interconnections required in light of the above-sampled anomalies; the connections they suggest are anomalous in respect to them. Hence the field that underlies and interconnects phenomena is not likely to be either the electromagnetic, the gravitational, or the strong or the weak nuclear fields. It is also not likely to be purely a conceptual construct, such as the (non-classical) probability fields of quantum mechanics. Rather, the indicated concept is likely to refer to a physically real field with novel, and possibly non-classical, properties.

## 1.3 THE FUNDAMENTAL VACUUM AS LOCUS OF THE INDICATED FIELD

The hypothesis advanced here postulates that the indicated space- and time-connecting field is an aspect or manifestation of the quantum vacuum. Here not the zero-point field (ZPF) as standardly interpreted is intended, but a fundamental field of which the ZPF is a specific manifestation. It is assumed that beyond the electromagnetic ZPF the fundamental vacuum has other, as yet incompletely understood, manifestations that generate, *inter alia*, the forces of inertia and gravitation, as well as the subtle forces that interconnect particles and systems built as integrated ensembles of particles in space and time.

The rationale for looking to the quantum vacuum as the locus of the interconnecting field can be spelled out. The cosmically extended vacuum is known to be the lowest energy state of a system of which the equations obey wave mechanics and special relativity. In an ontological interpretation it is considerably more than that, however. As Paul Dirac pointed out, all 'matter' is created out of this space-time pervading and, in itself, imperceptible substratum. At the threshold of $10^{27}$erg/cm$^3$ quantised particles arise from the vacuum pair-wise, with a positive-energy particle emerging into space-time and a negative-energy particle remaining in the field. The latter's energy density is estimated by John Wheeler to be $10^{94}$erg/cm$^3$; a quantity greater — some $10^{40}$ times greater, according to David Bohm — than the energy bound in matter in the observable universe.

Contemporary physics recognises the vacuum-origin of particles and has experimental proof of a variety of vacuum-particle interactions. For example, the ZPF of the vacuum is known to create a radiation pressure on two closely spaced metal plates: between the plates some wavelengths of the vacuum field are excluded, thereby reducing its energy density with respect to the field outside. This creates a pressure — known as the *Casimir Effect* — that pushes the plates inward and together. The ZPF is also known to act on the electrons that orbit atomic nuclei. Electrons 'jump' from one energy state to another, and the photons they emit exhibit the *Lamb-shift*, a frequency that, due to the presence of the ZPF, is slightly shifted from its normal value. Moreover it appears that stable atoms endure in space-time owing to interactions with the ZPF. The electron that orbits hydrogen atoms, for example, constantly radiates energy and would move progressively closer to the nucleus were it not that the quantum of energy it absorbs from the vacuum offsets the energy lost due to its orbital motion. Consequently the stability of hydrogen, as of other atoms in the universe, is due in part to interactions with the ZPF.

There may be quantum-vacuum interactions that mainstream theoretical physics does not as yet recognise, although some theoreticians have speculated on their occurrence. In 1968 Andrei Sakharov suggested that gravitation may be due to dynamic processes in the quantum vacuum in the presence of matter.[3] The hypothesis was further developed, first by János Lajossy, and then by László Gazdag, as a mathematical 'post-relativity theory'.[4] In this theory the vacuum is a physically real medium, unobservable in itself, but capable of producing observable effects. It has super-fluid properties, so that objects moving uniformly through it do not experience its presence, while non-uniform motion produces friction and hence observable effects. At speeds approaching the velocity of light, this gives rise to the relativistic infinities.

In the mid 1970s Paul Davies and William Unruh put forward a hypothesis based on the difference between uniform and accelerated motion in the vacuum. Uniform motion would exhibit the vacuum's spectrum as isotropic, whereas accelerated motion would produce a thermal radiation that breaks open the directional symmetry. The *Davies-Unruh Effect* prompted some physicists to investigate whether accelerated motion through the ZPF would produce incremental effects. This expectation has borne fruit.

### 1.4 INERTIA AND GRAVITATION AS PRODUCTS OF A SECONDARY VACUUM FIELD

A recent finding concerning vacuum interaction effects is the mathematical demonstration by Bernhard Haisch, Alfonso Rueda and Harold Puthoff that inertia may be a product of interaction between charged particles and the vacuum. In their treatment inertia appears as a vacuum-based Lorentz-force, originating at the subparticle level and creating opposition to the acceleration of material objects.[5] The accelerated motion of objects through the vacuum produces a magnetic field, and the particles that constitute the objects are deflected by this field. The larger the object the more particles it contains, hence the stronger the deflection and greater the inertia.

The interpretation proposed by Haisch, Rueda and Puthoff derives the inertial mass $m_i$ on the basis of the consideration that in stationary as well as in uniform-motion frames the interaction of a particle with the ZPF results in random oscillatory motion. Fluctuating charged particles produce a dipole scattering of the ZPF parametrised by the scattering spectral coefficient $h\,(w)$ that is frequency-dependent. Because of the relativistic transformations of the ZPF, in accelerated frames the interaction between a particle and the field acquires a direction: the 'scattering' of ZPF radiation generates a directional resistance force. This force is proportional to, and directed against, the acceleration vector for the subrelativistic case. It turns out to have the proper relativistic generalisation.[6]

However, if inertial mass originates in interaction between the ZPF and charged particles, then the principle of inertia-gravitation equivalence requires that gravitational mass should so originate as well. In that case gravitation becomes a force originating in ZPF-charge interactions, similar to Sakharov's interpretation. This hypothesis is cogent, even if the general relativistic treatment of gravitation as space-time curvature functions perfectly well: it is possible to show, namely, that there is an analytically equivalent interpretation according to which gravitation is a force generated by the motion of charged particles in the ZPF. The alternative interpretation is based on the consideration that the electric component of the ZPF causes charged particles to oscillate, and the oscillation gives rise to secondary electromagnetic fields. As a result a given particle experiences both the electric forces of the zero-point field, which causes it to oscillate, and the secondary forces that are triggered in the field by another particle. The secondary field generated by the second particle acts back on the first particle. The net effect is an attractive force among the two particles. Thus gravitation is a long-range interaction among particles, much as the *van der Waals force*.[7]

Given the principle of the equivalence of the inertial and the gravitational forces, vacuum/charged-particle interaction theories of inertia and gravitation stand or fall together. While they are not uncontroversial, their implications have much to commend them. For one thing, gravitation no longer appears as a mysterious force acting between two bodies distant and separate from one another in space and time. In classical physics this force constitutes a metaphysical 'action-at-a-distance', but in general relativity it is seen as mediated by the geometry of the space-time. While it is not clear how a geometrical structure can create or convey a physically real field, unless it is viewed as an ether-like space-time medium (a view to which Einstein himself inclined in his later years), we can now note that gravitation need not be given in that ether-like space-time medium. This eliminates a vexing anomaly, for if the staggering energy-density of the vacuum were associated with gravitation (through the relativistic-equivalence of energy and mass) all mass in the universe would instantly collapse to Planck dimensions. In the alternative ZPF/charge interaction theory this cannot occur: the vacuum does not act upon itself. Gravitation is not given in the zero-point field in the absence of matter; it is only created by the motion of charged particles. Hence its value is limited to the masses of these particles, rather than extending to the mass-equivalent of all the force particles (bosons) in the vacuum.[8]

It is noteworthy that mathematically elaborated attempts are now produced that trace inertia and gravitation, similarly to the Casimir Effect and the Lamb-shift, to interactions with the zero-point field of the vacuum. If this work treats a truly fundamental physical phenomenon, it must be seen as describing a general vacuum-reaction effect. The implication is the presence of a fundamental vacuum-based interactive field. Within the primary vacuum field, a secondary field appears to be generated, producing the phenomena of inertia and gravitation. The present hypothesis suggests that the secondary fields generated in the vacuum are not limited to the ZPF and its inertia and gravitation-creating effects, but includes a non-electromagnetic field of which the primary effect is to interlink particles across space and time. The postulation of the non-electromagnetic secondary vacuum field can account for a wider range of interconnected phenomena, including massively adaptive mutations in biology, and space- and time-transcending 'transpersonal' effects in the sphere of mind and consciousness.

## 2. The physical basis of the psi-field

Elementary particles are not classically discrete entities, but are embedded elements of the fundamental vacuum, much as solitons are embedded elements in a fluid with non-linear characteristics. The non-uniform motion of these particles breaks open the homogeneity and isotropy of the fundamental vacuum and produces secondary fields. In addition to the electromagnetic ZPF, these fields include the non-electromagnetic field we shall term *psi-field*. This consists not of classical electromagnetic (transverse) waves, but of interfering scalar (longitudinal) waves.[9] Trains of scalar waves interfere, and through the resulting *Schrödinger holograms* code information on the state and motion of the particles, and systems of particles, that were responsible for the waves.[10]

### 2.1. SPATIAL CONNECTIVITY THROUGH THE PSI-FIELD

Scalar waves are indicated in view of their potentially supraluminal velocity of propagation: this is required to account for the quasi-instanteity of some forms of interconnection. In a seminal paper published in 1903, E.T. Whittaker has shown that longitudinal waves such as scalars propagate with a finite velocity that may be greater than the speed of light. Propagation velocity is proportional to the mass-density of the medium in which the scalars occur. The vacuum's mass-density is the pertinent parameter: it defines the local electrostatic scalar potential. This is a variable quantity, higher in regions of dense mass, in or near stars and planets, and lower in deep space (a variation due to the increase in vacuum flux intensity by the accumulation of charged masses).[11] Consequently scalars travel faster through matter-dense regions of the vacuum than in deep space, much as longitudinally propagating sound waves travel faster in a dense medium than in a thin medium such as air.

Just as importantly, scalar wavefronts interfere, rather than pass through one another like classical electromagnetic waves. Interfering wavefronts code and convey information, similar to holograms. Consequently psi-field hypothesis states that the waves triggered in the vacuum by the motion of charged particles are scalar waves, and the patterns produced by them are Schrödinger holograms, made up of scalar interference patterns.

## 2.2. TRANSLATION BETWEEN SPACE-TIME MOTION AND THE PSI-FIELD

The interaction of charged particles, and ensembles of charged particles, with the scalar-structured secondary vacuum field can be mapped as a two-way Fourier transformation. The psi-field encodes the coefficients of the interfering scalar wavefronts produced by the motion of charged particles, and this information is decoded by particles and systems of particles in isomorphic states.

Particles move in relativistic space-time and obey general relativity laws. However, the scalars triggered by them in the psi-field propagate not in space-time, but in an underlying, essentially spectral domain similar to (although not identical with) Bohm's implicate order. Consequently the scalars created by the motion of particles in the field represent a translation from the spatio-temporal to the spectral domain: space-time motion is transformed into scalar interference patterns. In the inverse Fourier transform — from the spectral to the spatio-temporal domain — interference patterns in the psi-field feed back to the corresponding motion in space-time. (Here space-time motion is conceived as motion in a dynamic spatio-temporal — rather than purely conceptual — configuration space.) As the spectral-transforms of configured spatio-temporal motion feed back to analogously moving particles — or analogously configured ensembles of particles — the latter are 'informed' with their own spatio-temporally configured motion.

In a metaphorical yet apt expression, we can say that the forward Fourier transform — from space-time motion to psi-field — constitutes a *read-in* of the former in the latter; this results in the structuring of the fundamental vacuum with the scalar interference patterns of the psi-field. In the inverse Fourier transform these patterns feed back to particles and systems of particles in space-time in a process that approximates the *read-out* of the patterns by the corresponding particles and their ensembles.

### 2.3. TEMPORAL CONNECTIVITY THROUGH THE PSI-FIELD

The repeated observation that some forms of interconnection among particles and systems of particles persists over time implies that a 'memory factor' may be given is nature. In psi-field hypothesis the vacuum-trace of objects in maintained to be the pertinent factor. This is supported by experimental evidence. Vladimir Poponin and co-workers of the Institute of Biochemical Physics of the Russian Academy of Sciences, and subsequently at the Heartmath Institute in the USA, placed a sample of a DNA molecule into a temperature-controlled chamber and subjected it to a laser beam. They found that the electromagnetic field around the chamber exhibits a specific structure, more or less as expected. But they also found that this structure persists long after the DNA itself has been removed from the laser-irradiated chamber. The DNA's imprint in the field continues to be present even when the DNA itself is no longer there. Poponin and collaborators concluded that a new field structure has been excited from the physical vacuum. The field is extremely sensitive; it can be excited by a range of energies close to zero. The 'phantom effect' is a manifestation, they claim, of a hitherto overlooked vacuum substructure.[12]

If the vacuum-trace triggered in the vacuum by the motion of particles and systems of particles does not significantly attenuate over time, the 'information' fed back by it functions as memory: it connects the present of the particles, and systems of particles, with their past.

### 2.4. INTERACTION OF MACROSCALE SYSTEMS WITH THE PSI-FIELD

If the full range of anomalous intersystemic connections are to be accounted for, interaction with the psi-field cannot be limited to microscale systems of the order of Planck's constant. This enlarge-ment of the postulated vacuum interaction effects does not require a fundamental revision of current concepts in physics. Although in macroscale systems quantum-level fluctuations are damped out by large-scale regularities obeying dynamical laws, interaction with wave-interference patterns in the vacuum could nevertheless occur. First of all, it is known that in populations of particles Poincaré resonances are amplified. Secondly, in chaotic or near-chaotic states macroscale systems are highly initial-condition dependent. This represents a sensitivity to environmental fluctu-ations that may extend to subtle wave-patterns propagating in the vacuum.

Particles and systems of particles are sensitive primarily to their own psi-field-based wave-patterns. In the case of individual particles, sensitivity (and hence manifest interaction effect) is limited to the degrees of freedom defined by the quantum state. In the case of macroscale ensembles of particles, however, sensi-tivity is defined by the 3n-dimensional configuration-space of the system as a whole. According to psi-field hypothesis, in dynami-cally indeterminate states typical of chaos, macroscale systems are 'in-formed' with the psi-field based Fourier-transform of their own 3n-dimensional configuration-space.

The in-formation of macroscale systems with enduring scalar interference patterns isomorphic with their configuration-space means that microparticles and macroscale systems are ongoingly in-formed by their past. However, such in-formation is not neces-sarily limited to the past of the given entities themselves, as par-ticles and systems of particles may prove to be sensitive to psi-field wave-patterns that are not the waveform traces of their own motion but are isomorphic with these traces. In the event that a number of systems assume identical or quasi-identical 3n-dimen-sional configuration spaces, they will be sensitive to, and hence in-formed by, each others' psi-field-based traces. We may assume that if particle-states and system configuration-spaces are nearly identical, the in-formation conveyed through the psi-field will not distinguish between them. Consequently psi-field in-formation will produce non-locality among microparticles when particles that at one time assumed identical quantum states are split. Analogous connections will be produced among macroscale systems that occupy closely analogous configuration-spaces. Because of the supraluminal velocity of scalar wave-propagations, the connections will be quasi-instantaneous.

## 3. Transpersonal connections

In previous epochs interconnections that transcended the known bounds of space and time have attracted the attention primarily of mystics and metaphysicians. Since mid-century, however, also some scientists have set themselves the task of finding acceptable explanations. Among them are a fair number of *physicists* (the principle explicanda here include quantum-non-locality and the possibility of teleportation), some *biologists* (to be explained is the simultaneous emergence of order in various realms of nature), and some *psychologists* and *psychiatrists* (in view of the set of experiences denoted 'transpersonal'). In the latter regard the practice and experience of *physicians* and *healers*, including the distinguished members of the British Psionic Medical Society, furnish significant evidence.

### 3.1. THE TRANSPERSONAL DOMAIN OF CONSCIOUSNESS

Psychologists and psychiatrists, as well as students of meditative, physical, and ecstatic states of consciousness, find that persons in altered states of consciousness (ASCs) can access contents of consciousness that are not conveyed by the bodily senses. In such states anomalous images, utterances, items of knowledge, entire languages, even complex series of events can surface. Stanislav Grof investigated ASCs in almost 40 years of clinical practice and concluded that every process in the universe that can be objectively observed in the ordinary state of consciousness can be subjectively experienced in the altered state.[13] He suggested that the standard cartography of the mind needs to be completed with additional elements: to the standard 'biographic-recollective' domain of the psyche we should add a 'perinatal' and a 'transpersonal' domain.[14]

## 3.2. BRAIN/MIND CONNECTIONS THROUGH THE PSI-FIELD

Grof's findings call for explanation in terms consistent with findings in the new physics. Psi-field hypothesis, as noted by Grof himself, offers a good fit: it has a concept of both spatial and temporal interconnection. In regard to transpersonal phenomena the principal explicandum is temporal interconnection: the apparent ability to retrieve past experiences over the long term. Memory must extend not only through the experiences undergone by an individual him or herself, but also beyond. Such 'transpersonal' memory requires that the memory storage should be extrasomatic: it involves a process of encoding and decoding information in and from the psi-field. More exactly, it consists of the translation of scalar interference patterns between that secondary vacuum field and the subject's 3n-dimensional cerebral structure. The translation occurs when the dynamic pattern of structure and activity in the subject's brain matches an interference pattern present in the field. This pattern may be the trace of the cerebral activity of the subject him or herself, or it may be that of the cerebral activity of another person whose cerebral structure happens to be isomorphic with that of the subject.

The claim that long-term memories are retrieved from a holographically coded medium exhibits a good fit with observation. Since Karl Lashley's classic animal experiments it has been generally recognised that memory is not localised in brain tissue but is distributed over wide brain regions. According to Karl Pribram, the relevant brain regions approximate holographic receptor patches. Second, recall appears to have an associative property: whenever any fragment of a recorded information is presented to attention, that fragment acts as a memory address for the recovery of a wide range of associated information (consistently with the fact that in a hologram any small part includes the full set of recorded information). Third, recall consists of a complex set of data (visual, acoustic, and related memories), often in the form of time-varying sets of data ('moving-scene memories'), suggesting mechanisms similar to those of multiplex holography. Fourth, access-time in the brain is not related to the scanning-time of the stored experiences but is dependent mainly on the level of attention of the subject and the emotional intensity accompanying the recall.

In consequence psi-field hypothesis suggests that long-term memory involves the retrieval of information stored in wave-interference form in the ambient field. The transpersonal variety of recall is due, then, to the coincidence of the subject's cerebral structure with that of another person, whether near or distant, living or already dead. The effect surfaces due to the enhanced probability that the subject's cerebral structure matches that of another person. Such 'pattern-match probability' increases with the number of persons whose brain works in a closely analogous manner. A large number of cerebral activities of a given type makes it likely that one brain matches the waveform traces coded in the field by other person's. When one hits on a coinciding transform, one retrieves the corresponding aspect of that person's experience. In consequence the corresponding item of experience appears in one's own consciousness.

Match between the subject and another person appears to be 'hard-wired' in the case of some identical twins (the phenomenon of 'twin pain') and it appears capable of being induced by close personal ties (such as between mothers and sons, husbands and wives or lovers), as well as by intentionality (in purposively 'sending' thoughts or images in telepathic experiments).

### 3.3. IMPLICATIONS FOR PSIONIC MEDICINE

Transpersonal effects have significant implications for medicine, as shown by the experience and practice of the Psionic Medical Society. Through focusing the consciousness of the physician on the bodily states of the patient, aided by an organic sample (witness) from the latter, information is derived regarding his or her concurrent bodily condition. This enables the physician to diagnose malfunctions and prescribe remedies. Given the memory component of the information, past malfunctions (miasms), extending to progenitors and other individuals with matching bodily 3n-dimensional configuration spaces, can also be diagnosed and treated. The phenomenon conforms to a basic finding regarding transpersonal phenomena: the transmitted information is not limited by the known constraints of space and time. In psi-field hypothesis quasi-instant location-independent connectivity is accounted for by the supraluminal velocity of scalar wave-propagation in the secondary non-electromagnetic vacuum field, and the retrieval of information from the past is ensured by the temporal persistence of the wave interference patterns in that field.

A satisfactory exploration of the physical basis of Psionic phenomena requires further in-depth analysis. The here outlined psi-field hypothesis offers a cogent basis for research.

### 3.4. CONCLUSIONS

Phenomena that are anomalous for mainstream science suggest the existence of subtle yet effective spatial and temporal connections between real-world entities in all the principal realms of investigation: the physical, the biological, as well as the psychological. Accounting for the findings calls for a physical interconnecting medium: a field with the corresponding space- and time-transcending properties. Psi-field hypothesis postulates such a field. It notes that the interaction of particles with the fundamental vacuum creates interfering scalar wavefronts (Schrödinger holograms) which feed back to particles in the same or analogous quantum states, and to macroscale systems in the same or analogous 3n-dimensional configuration-spaces. In consequence particles that at one time occupied identical quantum states, and macroscale systems that at one time assumed analogous configuration-spaces, continue to be in-formed by their shared past. As the feedback occurs at speeds superior to the velocity of light, we obtain a physical basis for a number of anomalous interconnections, including those that link microparticles, living organisms, and the brain and consciousness of human beings.

## References

1. For a detailed account see Ervin Laszlo, *The Creative Cosmos*, Edinburgh, Floris Books 1993; *The Interconnected Universe*, Singapore and London: World Scientific 1995; *The Whispering Pond*, Rockport, Shaftesbury and Brisbane, 1996
2. Ervin Laszlo, Is there an interconnecting field? *Science Spectra* 5 (1998), 70–71
3. A. Sakharov, Vacuum quantum fluctuations in curved space and the theory of gravitation. *Soviet Physics – Doklamy*, 12, 11 (1968)
4. László Gazdag, *A Relativitás Elméleten Túl* (Beyond Relativity Theory). Szenci Molnár Társaság, Budapest, 1995; 'Superfluid mediums, vacuum spaces' *Speculations in Science and Technology*, Vol. 12,1,1989; and 'Combining of the gravitational and electromagnetic fields', *ibid.*, Vol. 16,1, 1993
5. Bernhard Haisch, Alfonso Rueda, and H.E. Puthoff, 'Inertia as a zero-point-field Lorentz force', *Physical Review A*, 49.2 (February 1994); Alfonso Rueda and Bernhard Haisch, 'Inertia as reaction of the vacuum to accelerated motion', *Physics Letters A*, 240 (30 March 1998)
6. Bernhard Haisch and Alfonso Rueda, 'The Zero-Point Field and the NASA Challenge to Create the Space Drive'. *Journal of Scientific Exploration* Vol. 11, No. 4 (Winter 1997)
7. The interpretation offered by Puthoff *et al.* consists of two parts. In the first part the energy of the ultrarelatavistic oscillations named *Zitterbewegung* by Schrödinger is equated to the gravitational mass $m_g$, after dividing by $c^2$. Except for a factor of 2, this produces a relationship between the gravitational mass and electrodynamical parameters identical to the above postulated inertial mass $m_i$. However, Puthoff *et al.* show that the gravitational mass $m_g$ should be reduced by a factor of 2, thereby achieving a strict equivalence between $m_i$ and $m_g$, i.e., between the forces of gravitation and inertia.

   The second part of Puthoff's analysis derives an inverse square force of attraction from the van der Waals force-like interaction between two driven oscillating dipoles. Admittedly this analysis is incomplete, requiring further theoretical development in the framework of a fully relativistic model.
8. In regard to inertia, the above attempts seek to derive the classical equations of motion from Maxwell's equations of electrodynamics, viewing inertia as a kind of electromagnetic drag force that is acceleration-dependent due to the spectral characteristics of the zero-point field. Here the stochastic electro-dynamics (SED) concept of the vacuum is pertinent, rather than the more usual quantum electrodynamics (QED) concept. However, work in progress suggests that discrepancies between SED and QED are not irremediable, so that the two approaches may one day be shown to generate identical results.
9. Further details are in the author's *The Interconnected Universe*, op. cit.
10. Scalars, unlike classical light and sound waves, do not satisfy D'Alembert's equation, of which the characteristic feature is the occurrence of a second time-derivative term of the wave amplitude. Generally such a term is a consequence of the inertial properties of matter. But in a massless force-field such as the

quantum vacuum these properties do not apply. Consequently vacuum waves can be represented by fundamental equations that contain only first-order time-derivative terms. There is only one kind of first-order time-derivative equations governing linear wave propagations and those are Schrödinger wave equations. cf. *The Interconnected Universe*, op. cit.

11  E.T. Whittaker, 'On the partial differential equations of mathematical physics', *Mathematische Annalen*, 57 (1903), 333–355

12. P. Gariaev and V.P. Poponin, 'Vacuum DNA phantom effect in vitro and its possible rational explanation', *Nanobiology* (1995)

13. Stanislav Grof, *The Adventure of Self-discovery*, Albany: The State University of New York Press, 1988

14. Stanislav Grof, *The Adventure of Self-discovery*, op. cit., xvi

# Orthodox Medicine — From Philosophical System to Science

*'The philosopher must begin with Medicine, and the physician must end with philosophy.'*

**Aristotle**

P sionic Medicine is predominantly an energy-based approach. It is, however, thoroughly based upon orthodox medicine. It is important to appreciate this, because it is not an alternative view, but an extension of the subject into the field of energetics. It is entirely appropriate, therefore, to consider the development of orthodox medicine from its origins as a philosophical system to its current scientific basis.

## A brief history of medicine

From time immemorial man has devised ways of caring for the sick by basing his treatments upon beliefs current at the time. From archaeological evidence we know that primitive man believed life to be ruled by both benevolent and hostile spirits. Illness or disease was attributed to demonic possession, and was treated by magical rites, the wearing of amulets and charms, and sometimes by primitive attempts at *trephination* — the boring of a hole in the skull — in order to let out the evil spirits.

Later, when man eventually gave up his nomadic existence as a hunter and food gatherer, he settled on the land and began to grow crops. As he became intimately involved with the process of nurturing his crops, he would inevitably realise that three factors were necessary to grow food — heat from the sun, water and earth. One can thus easily imagine how the early settlers would deify these requisites of plant life to form a basic cosmology or theory of the universe. To these three he would add the invisible cosmic element of air, or breath in order to account for the special needs of both man and animals.

And so, we can see how a theory of the *Elements — Earth, Air, Fire* and *Water* — could have developed to explain the nature of the universe. However, it would not account for the fact that plants and animals are different from the rest of the inanimate world. In order to allow for this, he would develop the concept of some form of Vital Force or energy.

Anthropology tells us that this simple philosophical blueprint has recurred across the globe throughout the centuries. The ancient Greeks refined it in the fifth century BC. Hippocrates of Cos, often referred to as the Father of Medicine, developed the idea that the four Elements acted upon by the Vital Force became activated into *humours* or *Vital Fluids* once they had been assimilated and absorbed into the body.

There were four Vital Fluids — *Blood, Phlegm, Black Bile* and *Yellow Bile*.

He taught that Air absorbed through the lungs would be transformed into Blood; Water would eventually become Phlegm; Earth (from the substance of food) would become Black Bile; and Heat or Fire would become Yellow Bile.

Aristotle added to this theory the idea of the Elements being linked to the *Four Qualities of Hot, Dry, Cold* and *Wet*. Each Element was conceived as being a mixture of two paired Qualities. This postulate allowed for the transformation of one Element into another, if the predominance of one Quality was altered. For example, Fire which is Hot and Dry, plus Water which is Cold and Wet, could respectively lose Dryness and Coldness to form Earth, which is Cold and Dry, and Air, which is Wet and Hot.

The second-century physician, Claudius Galen, further refined this theory by linking the Vital Fluids (or humours) and Qualities with the tissues of the body. From this arose the further idea that the Vital Fluids could be linked to the Temperaments of Man. There were thought to be four basic Temperaments — Sanguine, Phlegmatic, Melancholic and Choleric. In addition, because these were also associated with paired Qualities, a predominance of one of the pairs would result in a further four sub-types, as well as one which would be a perfect balance of all four Qualities. Hence, nine constitutional types of people or nine temperaments were recognised (Figure 3).

Of the four basic temperaments the pure Choleric temperament was generally thought to be confident, irascible, touchy and proud. The Phlegmatic or Lymphatic temperament was fussy, a bit obsessional, practical, but tended to shun the limelight. The Sanguine temperament was excitable, impressionable, impulsive

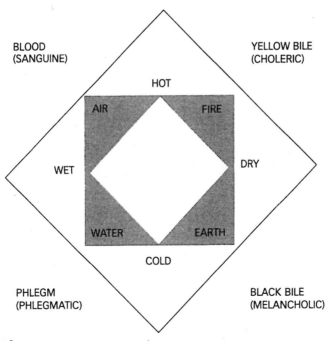

Figure 3

and sometimes unreliable. The Melancholic temperament was cautious, serious, industrious and solitary, and with a tendency to become depressed.

It also came to be believed that different organs were influenced by one of three *Essences* or *Spirits*. The heart was thought to be the site of the *Vital Spirit*, which was responsible for hope, humanity, morality, and courage. The liver was thought of as the site of *Natural Spirit*, which nourished the body. Finally, the brain was associated with *Animal Spirit*, which gave the individual imagination, judgement and memory.

Astrological influences were also considered important, since it was thought that both the Vital Fluids and the Essences were influenced by both the Zodiacal signs and the planets.

Health was thus considered to be dependent upon a balance between the Vital Fluids, disease being the inevitable consequence of any imbalance. Treatment involved restoring the balance by reducing the *peccant* or disease-producing humour. For example, if blood was conceived to be the offending humour, then bloodletting would restore the balance. Our word *exsanguinate*, meaning to drain of blood, can be seen to originate from such practice; similarly, *cholagogues*, remedies which affected the flow of bile; *emetics*, which caused vomiting; and *purgatives* which cleared out the bowel, were all used to remove other excessive peccant humours.

Another method of restoring balance was by utilising the *Doctrine of Contraries*. This meant that a predominantly *Moist* disease could be cured by administering a *Dry* remedy, whereas a *Hot Drug* would be most effective against a *Cold disease*. This system of pharmacology became known as *Galenism*, after the physician Galen, and the drugs came to be known as *Galenicals*.

Many Galenicals were extremely complicated, consisting of numerous ingredients of dubious value. Galen himself frequently prescribed remedies consisting of as many as one hundred ingredients. The substances used ranged from the magico-medical (pulverised Egyptian mummy foot), to the exotic (ground unicorn or rhinoceros horn), to the commonplace plants and herbs.

Indeed, in our expression 'as cool as a cucumber' we see a reference to the use of this simple vegetable as a Galenical. It is a cooling agent, which has been found to have a scientific rationale, since it is rich in salicylates, which are of course related to aspirin.

This rather simplified description of how man could arrive at a theory of elements leading onto a humoral theory serves as a blueprint for a philosophical explanation of medicine. By observing the universe and deducing how he develops from the basic building blocks of the elements, man would logically come to believe that the human body represents the universe in miniature. In addition, he would naturally conceive that the same laws that govern the universe regulate health. Thus, man the *microcosm* reflects the universe, the *macrocosm*.

## The birth of scientific medicine

The humoral theory as outlined above was the dominant theory of Medicine in the West until the Renaissance, when the birth of the scientific approach seemingly made nonsense of the concepts of Hot, Cold, Moist and Dry conditions.

In 1543, three books were simultaneously published in Europe, which were to rock the medical and scientific world. These were: *De Humani Corporis Fabrica* (*The Anatomical Drawings of Andreas Vesalius*); the first translation of the *Greek Mathematics and Physics of Archimedes*; and Nicolaus Copernicus' *De Revolutionibus Orbium Coelestium* (*The Revolution of the Heavenly Orbs*). With these works came the realisation that diseases could be linked to anatomical structure; that physical events were measurable and predictable according to mathematical laws; and that the system of astrology was based upon the fallacious belief that the stars and planets were fixed in positions according to their astrological roles. The Scientific Revolution had started and objective observation and measurement began to replace tradition and the word of written authority.

One of the main advocates of the new approach was Santorio Santorio, a friend and contemporary of Galileo, who in 1625 demonstrated that the temperature of a Hot- predominant individual and a Cold-predominant person was likely to be the same.[1]

Three years later, in 1628, the scientific method was given a further boost when William Harvey published his monogram *De Motu Cordis et Sanguinis in Animalibus* (*On the Motion of the Heart and Blood in Animals*). By substantiating theory with experimental proof he laid the foundations of the science of physiology.

## Dualism

At roughly the same time, René Descartes (1596–1650), a mathematician and philosopher, was laying down the ground plan for what was to become known as Cartesian philosophy. Unconvinced by tradition and theological dogma, he sought a mechanistic explanation of every phenomenon. He believed that nature worked according to mechanical laws, and that the human body was a complicated machine designed by God and infused with a *'rational soul'*. Also, since he did not believe that animals had a rational soul, but could be thought of as sophisticated automatons, the workings of the organs of the body could, he claimed, be legitimately studied by animal experimentation.

Because of this mind–body dualism inherent in the Cartesian approach — the doctrine that mind and body were separate entities — it became possible for researchers to compartmentalise the two, so that the study of Medicine became the study of man's inner workings. For this reason, the flood of discoveries about physiology led onto the belief that illness could eventually be explained entirely in terms of mechanistic principles. Indeed, following the Italian Giovanni Battista Morgagni's (1682–1771) demonstration that disease could be localised to particular organs by correlating post-mortem reports with clinical case-records, the new science of pathology came into being. Effectively, the point was reached when the disease rather than the patient became the target of Medicine.

The influence of the Christian Church has to be alluded to here, for it was about this time that it began to permit the dissection of human corpses for scientific investigation. The importance of this is that the Church saw in mind–body dualism a reaffirmation of its own standing. In other words, the body, being a weak and imperfect vessel which temporarily housed the soul, was a suitable subject for study by mere scientists, whereas the study of the mind and soul belonged rightly to the Church. Thus, with the blessing of the Church, the mind–body dualism furthered the way for the establishment of the biomedical model of Medicine. Increasing knowledge about structure and function seemed to reaffirm the notion that the body was a machine, that disease was a consequence of malfunction of parts of the machine, and that the role of the doctor was to repair the mechanism.

## The biomedical model of Western orthodox medicine

From then on, diseases were classified according to disturbed pathology, and further 'pathological sciences' came into being. Thus, just as the basic medical sciences had been extended to include anatomy, histology, physiology and biochemistry, their pathological counterparts became morbid anatomy, histopathology, morbid physiology and chemical pathology.

On the clinical side, because physicians were no longer seeking indicators of humoral imbalance, but were aiming to elicit visual and auditory signs of malfunction, there followed a spate of diagnostic inventions. Réné-Théophile-Hyacinthe Laënnec's (1781–1826) invention of the stethoscope permitted doctors to listen to the flow of air in the lungs, the beat of the heart, and the sound of the intestines. Similarly, Hermann von Helmholtz's (1821–1894) invention of the ophthalmoscope allowed an inspection of the interior of the eye. In the 1820s an aural speculum for examination of the ear was perfected, and in 1896 Scipione Riva-Rocci produced the first effective sphygmomanometer for the measurement of blood pressure. All of these instruments, or slightly more sophisticated versions, are to be found in the medical bag of virtually every general medical practitioner today.

In 1895, Wilhem Conrad Röntgen (1845–1922) discovered the

amazing phenomenon of the X-ray. Because it was realised that these rays could penetrate almost any material and produce a photographic shadow, their use in medicine was quick to follow.

Shortly after this Henri Becquerel (1852–1909) discovered the radioactive element uranium. This is turn was followed in 1898 by the isolation of radium from pitchblende by Pierre (1859–1906) and Marie Curie (1867–1934). From these great discoveries began the respective disciplines of radiology and radiotherapy.

The name of Louis Pasteur (1822–1895) stands out in nineteenth-century medicine, for he effectively established the field of bacteriology when he elaborated his *germ theory of disease*. For the first time physicians began to understand the nature of infections, and could start to use precautions to prevent their spread. Following him, Robert Koch (1843–1910) discovered the tuberculosis bacillus, one of the major killers of the day.

These two men undoubtedly dominated the early days of bacteriology, but after Pasteur's death further research split into two main directions. In Germany, under Koch's lead, bacteriologists set about discovering and cataloguing the organisms responsible for various infectious illnesses. In France, following Pasteur's work on vaccination, the emphasis was placed on understanding the mechanisms of immunity.

The Russian, Elie Metchnikoff (1845–1916), added to our understanding of immunity when he demonstrated that certain white blood cells were capable of destroying bacteria by engulfing them (the process of phagocytosis), while others could develop antibodies against future bacterial invasion. For this he was awarded the Nobel Prize in 1908.

An important discovery was made by Pierre-Paul-Émile Roux (1853–1933), a protégé of Pasteur, when he reported finding a disease-causing agent which was so small that it was ultra-microscopic and capable of passing through even the finest of filters. Thus were *viruses* first discovered, opening up another new discipline of virology.

Subsequent to this, micro-organisms of other sizes were discovered. Howard Taylor Ricketts (1871–1910) working in the USA discovered a group of organisms which were intermediate in size between bacteria and viruses, and which caused conditions like Rocky Mountain Spotted Fever. This important group — *rickettsia* – was named after him.

## The search for the magic bullet — pharmacology joins the lists

For many centuries mercury in the form of calomel (mercurous chloride) was used in huge, toxic and often fatal doses to treat syphilis. In 1909 Paul Ehrlich (1854–1915) and Sahachiro Hata (1873–1938) developed the drug *salvarsan*, also called 606, because it was actually produced at the six hundred and sixth attempt. It was a compound of arsenic and completely supplanted the use of mercury. It was the first truly effective drug against an infective illness and it led Ehrlich to believe that there were other 'magic bullets' waiting to be found to cure diseases.

It was not until 1932, however, that the next major advance took place, when *prontosil*, the forerunner of the sulphonamide antibiotics, was produced. These drugs had a dramatic effect in the treatment of pneumonia, but they had significant problems. Then in 1940, partly driven by the necessities of war, Ernst Chain (1906–1979) and Howard Florey (1898–1968) published work on the use of penicillin in the treatment of infection. Their work was, of course, based upon the earlier anti-bacterial effect of the penicillium mould by Alexander Fleming (1881–1955) in 1928. All three were awarded the Nobel Prize in 1945.

The later years of the twentieth century saw an explosion of discoveries in the field of pharmacology as such drugs as insulin, steroids and other analgesic and anti-inflammatory agents came into use. And because of this, together with advances in other disciplines like immunology, it has been possible to develop life-saving techniques such as dialysis and organ transplantation.

## Psychiatry — the medicine of the mind

Earlier in this chapter it was inferred that René Descartes was ultimately responsible for the doctrine of mind–body dichotomy, which effectively resulted in removing the mind from any consideration of the disease process. Fortunately, as we shall see later, this attitude is changing dramatically within the western model of orthodox medicine.

The conventional treatment of mental illness in the early eighteenth century was a disgrace. So-called *'lunatics'* were incarcerated in asylums and treated little better than prisoners. Enlightenment did not arrive until 1798 when Phillipe Pinel struck off the shackles of the patients at the Asylum Bicêtre in France.

In 1870, Henry Maudsley published a book on the relationship between mind and body in the causation of mental illness. It was a brilliant book for the time and was to pave the way for a greater understanding of the mind in the twentieth century.

Current psychiatry basically consists of three streams of practice. These are: psychotherapy, behavioural psychiatry and organic psychiatry.

The dominant stream at the beginning of the twentieth century was undoubtedly the approach developed by Sigmund Freud (1856–1939) and his two leading collaborators, Carl Gustav Jung (1875–1961) and Alfred Adler (1870–1937).

Freud, by first using hypnosis, taught that certain mental disorders were the result of unresolved conflicts buried deep within the unconscious mind. He described various mental mechanisms, which seemed to be involved in both normal life and in neurotic states, examples being repression, forgetting and symbolisation. He conceptualised the mind as having three main components — the *id*, *super-ego* and *ego*, and developed the famous technique of psychoanalysis by free association.

Adler and Jung, both disciples of Freud, also used psychoanalytical techniques, yet they thought that Freud laid too much emphasis on sexual frustration as a cause of neurosis. Adler stressed the need for self-esteem, and Jung that of the search for self-fulfilment. Jung, of course, became famous for his concept of the *collective unconscious* and his description of psychological archetypes. Each of them went their separate way, the result being the founding of three schools of psychoanalytic thought.

Behavioural psychiatry, the second stream of thought, had its origins in the work of the Russian Ivan Pavlov (1849–1936), who was awarded the Nobel Prize in 1904 for his work on the digestive system. In later life he had turned his attention to mental disorder, and by applying his concept of the *conditioned reflex* he was responsible for establishing the behaviourist school of thought. Thus, mental illness could be attributed to learned behaviour, which could be treated by 'unlearning' the conditioned response.

The organic approach essentially subscribes to the view that mental activity is a product of brain function, thereby meaning that aberrant mental activity is a result of organic (i.e., physical or chemical) changes within the brain. Treatment then consists of the use of psychotropic drugs, electro-convulsive therapy (ECT) or 'psychosurgery'.

This is, of course, a gross oversimplification, because virtually all doctors are now aware of the importance of psychological factors in every patient's perception of their illness.

## Modern medicine and surgery

The advances, which have taken place in both medicine and surgery throughout the twentieth century, are legion. The control of pain, better understanding of blood coagulation, fluid and electrolyte balance, infection control and anaesthetic technology have made our operating theatres places where the most incredible procedures can be performed. Many of the major organs can now be transplanted, traumatically amputated limbs can feasibly be replanted, and hip and knee joints are now routinely replaced. Not only that, but with laparoscopes and fibre optics surgeons are now pushing back the frontiers by developing minimally invasive surgery, or 'keyhole surgery' as it is more popularly known.

On the medical side, drugs are being developed all the time which specifically target receptor sites to produce effects on single organs or systems. Peptic ulceration can now be treated medically rather than surgically as was often the case but three decades ago. Many cancers which had appalling mortality rates now have realistic chances of survival, if not cure. Hormonal treatments have advanced considerably, so that women can now plan their families, and at a later age pass through the menopause with reduced risk of osteoporosis, bone fractures and heart disease.

In the early twentieth-century hospital doctors could become general physicians or general surgeons. That is, it was possible for one man to cover all of the disciplines within medicine or surgery. As medical technology has advanced, however, and the body of knowledge has increased, so too has the need for specialisation, and for sub-specialisation.

Critics of orthodox medicine would aver that the reductionism, which causes sub-specialisation (which is really super-speciali-sation), results in doctors only being interested in their field, in the part of the body to which their speciality relates. This is naïve, however, because specialisation of necessity leads to teamwork. And it is teamwork that nowadays leads to advancement in science.

In the last third of the twentieth century, the specialities in a sense began to cross-specialise. Inevitably, there would be areas of mutual interest, since no system of the body can really be viewed in isolation from others. For example, since the heart can not be viewed merely as a pump, but as a pump with innervation, some researchers would specialise in neuro-cardiology. Similarly, work would be done on such subjects as immunopsychiatry, neuroendocrinology, neuropsychology and psychophysiology.

Essentially, one can liken it to making a tapestry. Each thread (each discipline) is an important and integral part of the whole, yet can only create a very limited effect on its own. At points where the thread crosses another (discipline) there are areas of mutual interest and a bit more effect is created. The more crossovers, the closer one gets to the picture and the overall effect that the individual threads cannot give alone. The end result of reductionism, in a sense, must be a move towards holism.

## Holistic medicine

Jan Smuts, the first Prime Minister of South Africa in his book *Holism and Evolution* first coined the term 'holism' in 1926. Decades later, in the 1960s, partly as a reaction towards the increasingly reductionist direction of modern medicine, and partly because of a growing public interest in Eastern philosophies, it became adapted as a desirable approach towards medicine. Essentially, it was a view that mind, body, spirit and the environment should all be taken into account in the health of the individual.

One means of studying this was through looking at systems and systems theory. Systems theory had been written about by Weiss[2] and Von Bertalanffy,[3] but it was George Engel,[4] Professor of Psychiatry at Rochester, New York, who applied it to health and illness. Engel pointed out that each system is at the same time a component of a higher system. For example, a cell is part of a tissue and tissue forms part of an organ, and so on. In other words, nothing exists in isolation. There is a place for examining the cell, but it has to be remembered that it is not isolated from the whole. It is like examining a fish out of water: it will give little information about the way it reacts with its environment, how it feeds, breathes, lives and dies. One has to study all the interacting systems. Engel was thus calling for a new model of medicine.

Indeed, with cross-specialisation already taking place, researchers were already accepting the role of the mind in health and illness (that is in *all* illness, not merely in illness of the mind, the domain of psychiatry), so the time was right for the further development of holistic medicine.

## Psychoneuroimmunology

In the 1960s, psychiatrist Dr George Solomon observed that certain women with particular personality traits, including passivity, and a tendency to long-suffering, were more prone to rapid progression of rheumatoid arthritis. Also was the observation that rats with implanted tumour cells were more likely to die quickly if they were subjected to stress. Solomon believed that somehow the mind was affecting the immune system, so he called the new field of study *psychoimmunology*.

In the 1970s psychologist Robert Ader made another amazing discovery. He found that rats could be conditioned to depress their immune systems. Working with Nicholas Cohen, an immunologist, they demonstrated that certain nerve pathways were likely to be in operation between the brain and the immune system, and that conditioning could affect the system. Accordingly, they expanded the name of the discipline to Psychoneuroimmunology (PNI). Neuroscientist Karen Bulloch later demonstrated that they were correct in their surmise, when she traced direct nerve pathways between the brain and the immune system.

Up to then it was known that nerve transmission provided a link between brain and immune system, but there was more to come. Candace Pert, a neuroscientist who discovered the opiate receptor, has performed extensive research to demonstrate that there are many chemicals produced in the body which feed back between brain and immune system. Indeed, she and her team have found that there are many receptor sites for these *neurotransmitters*, or *informational molecules*[5] and that these are not limited to the brain and central nervous system. There are sites on both red and white blood cells, stomach and kidney. Because of these, one can see how the body can react to stress so swiftly.

So far, over 65 of these neurotransmitters have been catalogued. These act literally like emotion-transmitters, in that when we feel a particular emotion, for example, anger, fear or jealousy, then a specific hormone or neurotransmitter is released throughout the fluid compartments of the body. Wherever it meets an appropriate receptor site, it will latch on, then enter the cell to affect its function.

Because we are now aware of both a neurological basis and a hormonal mechanism whereby the mind can affect the body, the discipline is sometimes referred to as Psychoneuroendocrinoimmunology

(PNEI). Whatever the name, its discoveries are proving of great value in our understanding of the way mind and body interact.

Two fascinating phenomena are worth mentioning. First is the fact that many people are able to delay their illness. This is often seen in people who manage to struggle through a heavy workload, then develop an illness on the first day of their holiday. Second is the observation that a disproportionate number of people die on their birthday or after some important anniversary or thing that they feel they have to do. William Shakespeare is a noted example of someone dying on his birthday. Why does it happen?

## Summary

This is a significant chapter because it is important to understand the way in which orthodox medicine has developed. It started as a philosophical system, then under the influence of Cartesian dualism advanced in a reductionist manner to delve deeper and deeper into the workings of the physical body, almost eliminating the mind from any consideration, except as a separate phenomenon, a separate area of study. However, with the recognition of holism and growing interest in systems theory there has come a realisation that mind, body and environment cannot be viewed in isolation.

Psychoneuroimmunology is now showing us how the mind and body interact, at least at the phenomenological level. This is of overwhelming importance, for it shows us how, if not why, the mind and body interact in health and illness. Yet it leaves us tantalisingly short of understanding ever more subtle causes of illness.

Psionic Medicine is the branch of medicine which is going to permit us to tap into those subtle realms. It is important to understand that it is not an alternative medicine in any sense. It is firmly based upon orthodox medicine, and upon all of the disciplines which make up orthodox medicine. It is a means whereby the subtle causes of illness can be delineated and removed, so that the underlying processes which cause the illness can be, if it is possible, halted in their track.

[1] This idea that Hot and Cold were to do with temperature was a misconception, however. The concepts of Hot and Cold should really have been regarded as metaphorical terms. Indeed, this is precisely how they have been regarded in the cultures, which still extensively practise medicine based upon a humoral theory.

[2] Weiss, P., The System of Nature and the Nature of Systems. In: *Towards a Non-centred Medical Science*, New York, Futura Pub. Co 1977

[3] Von Bertalanffy, L., *General Systems Theory*, New York, Braziller, 1968

[4] Engel, G., The Need For a New Medical Model; the challenge of biomedicine, *Science* 196:129-136, 1976

[5] See Candace Pert's book *The Molecules of Emotion*, Pocket Books, Simon & Schuster, London, 1997

# Subtle Bodies and Psionic Medicine

*'Man is what he is by virtue of body, etheric body, soul (astral body), and ego (spirit). He must in health be seen and understood from the aspects of these his members; in disease he must be observed in the disturbance of the equilibrium; and for his healing we must find the remedies that can restore that balance.'*

**Fundamentals of Therapy,**
**Rudolph Steiner**

In the last chapter we considered the development of medicine from its origins as a philosophical system through years of increasing reductionism and mind–body duality, until it reached its current acceptance of the interaction between mind, body and immune system. This illustrates that it is at least, if not at last, on the right track. In this chapter we are going to consider how the capstone of our pyramid of medicine can be added by looking at the energetic side of man.

## More than flesh and blood

Virtually all cultures have believed that man is more than a physical body organised by a strange, wrinkled organ — the brain — within the skull. Almost without exception they have come to the conclusion that some vitalising force, spirit or soul resides within the body and that at death this subtle energy or soul leaves the body, usually to travel to some other realm.

.Some societies have taken this basic idea further and conceptualised different 'layers' to man, in both the physical and the subtle sense.

## The ancient Egyptians

The ancient Egyptians are often thought of as a race obsessed with death. This is a misconception that has arisen simply because of the funerary artefacts and monumental works which they left behind. In fact, they were a people who loved life and hoped for a continuation of it in another realm of being. Their religious practices, however, led them to believe that the personality had to be kept as intact as possible if they were to pass the tests before the gods in the Hall of Judgement.

In pre-dynastic days the early Egyptians believed that the three important constituents of the individual were the body, the soul and the spirit. As their religion became ever more complex, however, they conceived of ever deeper layers of being which constituted the personality, all of which had to be protected if the individual was to enjoy the after-life with Osiris in the Happy Fields. Different papyri tell us of different combinations, but in total there were ten layers or aspects of the personality, as follows: *Sahu* (cosmic body), *Ka* (energy double of the physical body), *Ba* (spirit double), *Khaibit* (shadow), *Khu* (spirit body), *Khat* (physical body), *Hati* (the physical heart), whose etheric counterpart was the *Ab* (heart or conscience), *Sekhem* (vital force) and *Ren* (name).

Let us focus on the Ka for a moment. This energetic double of the person was thought able to leave the body during sleep, so that it could wander about and visit people and places, those journeys and meetings surviving within the memory. Thus dreams were explained as being actual Ka experiences, whereby the dreamer's Ka would be conceived as having met the Ka or having seen the physical form of another individual on one of its travels.

Yet it was not only the human being that was thought to have a Ka. Everything that existed was thought to have a Ka — birds, animals, fish, plants, trees and inanimate objects. Thus, when a man ate, the physical food nourished his Khat, his body, but the Ka of the food nourished the Ka that was part of him.

It is easy to dismiss the Egyptians as being philosophically or theologically naïve, yet there is great sophistication in their conception of the nature of man.

## The ancient Greeks

The ancient Greeks were, of course, a highly sophisticated and intelligent people much concerned with the nature of the universe and of man's place within it. Empedocles, a native of Agrigentum in Sicily, who flourished around 450BC, postulated that the universe was composed of four elements – Earth, Air, Fire and Water, which were governed by the forces of love and hate, or attraction and repulsion. Accordingly, it came to be believed that the matter of the universe, and therefore man as well, was made up of these elements.

The Neoplatonic view, which was essentially a synthesis of Platonism, Aristotlism and Pythagoreanism, considered that the individual had five main components. These were the *soma*, the physical body; the *psyche*, which was the individual's personality, a sort of lower mind; the *thymos*, the active, rational and mortal aspect of man; the *pneuma*, or vital energy and vital air; and the *nous*, the higher or divine mind, beyond which was deity itself. At the time of death the thymos expired, allowing the psyche release to travel to the underworld to enjoy the after-life. Essentially, the thymos and psyche were two aspects of being, corresponding to the Ka and Ba of the ancient Egyptians.

## The Eastern concept

Hinduism is the last main polytheistic religion practised on Earth. Although it has no fixed scriptural canon, the spiritual doctrines are to be found in the *Vedas* (literally meaning 'knowledge'), a collection of ancient hymns and teachings, apparently given to the *rishis* (seers) by Lord Brahma, the creator. They were written between 1500BC and 500BC.

Within the Vedas there are descriptions of the physical and subtle nature of man. Essentially, it is stated that there are several layers, levels or bodies existing at one and the same time, which are linked by subtle anatomical features including the *chakras* (energy centres) and the *nadis* (energy channels).

In the tenth century the Guru Goraknath wrote the *Gorakshashatakam*, a treatise on chakra awakening and meditation. In the sixteenth century an even more comprehensive account was written by Purananda Svami, in *Shri-Tattva-Cintamini*.

Tibetan Buddhist texts also describe these subtle bodies and chakric system. There are differences between them, yet they can be seen as overlaps in interpretation.

## The Theosophical movement

In the late 1870s, Madame Helena Petrovna Blavatsky (1831–1891) co-founded the *Theosophical Society* with Colonel Harry Steel Olcott, in Madras, India. The term comes from the Greek words *theos*, meaning 'god', and *sophia*, meaning 'wisdom'. According to the movement's teachings, all religions stem from a common root of ancient wisdom, which can be discerned from the common myths and symbols which abound, and that a study of them will lead to truth and spiritual unity. Within this framework man is conceived of as a spiritual being, and that there are seven spheres of consciousness, or seven subtle bodies. A central tenet of theosophy is the concept of karma-governed reincarnation.

## Rudolph Steiner and Anthroposophy

Rudolph Steiner (1861–1925), an Austrian philosopher, artist, scientist and educationalist, had been developing his own ideas about the spiritual nature of man, partly through his clairvoyant experiences and his ability to access the Akashic Records,[1] when he first came to the attention of the theosophists. His lectures proved to be very popular, and in 1902 he founded a German branch of the Theosophical Society.

Steiner's views were markedly different from the theosophists, however. Whereas the dominant influence in theosophy had been the philosophies of the East, Steiner's orientation was pre-eminently Western. By 1913 he broke away to found his own organisation, the *Anthroposophical Society*. The term, coming from the Greek *anthropos*, meaning 'man', and *sophia*, meaning 'wisdom', shows the different emphasis of his ideas.

Anthroposophy covers a whole range of activities, including spiritual science, religion, education, organic agriculture and health. Indeed, a whole system of medicine, anthroposophical medicine, developed utilising his guiding principles.

Steiner taught that there was a fourfold nature of man. This he had been personally aware of through his own psychic ability. Effectively, he believed that there were four bodies which made up the individual, these being:

- Physical body
- Etheric body — the energy double which exerted 'formative forces' upon the physical
- Astral body — the knowing emotional body, which contained the individual's drives and motivations
- Ego — the self-consciousness, soul and spirit

As mentioned in Chapter One, Steiner's concept of the subtle bodies and the interaction between them had a profound influence upon Dr George Laurence. He came to believe that the cause of many illnesses must arise from somewhere other than the physical body. The etheric body seemed to be such a possible source.

## The subtle bodies

From our discussion so far, we can see that there are many similarities in the systems that we have considered. An amalgamation of them all is broadly accepted as being as follows:

- Physical body — the equivalent of the ancient Egyptian Khat, the Greek Soma

- Etheric body — the energetic body which contains the organising and regulating mechanisms which effectively control the body's functions from the atomic level upwards. The equivalent of the Ancient Egyptian Ka, the Greek Psyche
- Astral body — a psychic body, the emotional body containing all emotional drives, passions. The equivalent of the ancient Egyptian Ba, the Greek Thymos
- Mental body — the body of thoughts or intellect
- Causal body — the higher self. In some interpretations there are yet higher levels leading to the absolute soul of the individual

These subtle bodies are perceived as different planes of being, and for this reason are probably better thought of as fields, rather than bodies (but from convention, we shall continue to refer to them as 'bodies'). They are all active in every one of us, but we are simply not conscious of them, mainly because we live in the physical realm and have senses limited to that realm. Having said that, most people are able to become aware of some of the lower levels with practice. It is not a case of discovering new talents, merely rediscovering dormant or forgotten talents. Indeed, rediscovering some of these dormant talents is fundamental to the practice of Psionic Medicine.

### Auras

Everyone has an *aura*, a multi-dimensional energy field, which is made up of the different subtle bodies. Sometimes these are described as being in actual layers, like the colours of a rainbow, being present around the body like a set of transparent, coloured Russian dolls. In fact, this is open to interpretation, because the word 'see' needs to be modified. One does not actually see an aura in the way that one sees a physical phenomenon. The aura is perceived when one allows one's 'conscious' to 'slip', or partially go to sleep. This is why people usually fail to see them. They are simply trying too hard to focus on a phenomenon which is a perception that is only in part visual.

People who see auras usually report them in ways that are unique to themselves. Also, the aura is not a static thing, but is constantly changing, reflecting the dynamic nature of the individual, of the life force of that person.

There is an extensive body of research and literature regarding auras. Walter J. Kilner, a physician at St Thomas's Hospital just before the Great War, discovered that an aura could be seen when the body was looked at through a dicyanin lens. His early researches were published in his book *The Human Aura* in 1911. Although it was greeted with much scepticism at the time, it did attract the attention of many eminent scientists, among them Sir Oliver Lodge.[2] By 1919, he formulated a system of auric diagnosis. In 1937 Oscall Bagnall, a Cambridge biologist, published his work *The Origin and Properties of the Human Aura.* Harold Saxton Burr did extensive research upon it as he came up with his L-field hypothesis. Hiroshi Motoyama in Japan and Valerie Hunt at the UCLA both conducted electromagnetic testing on chakras and subtle bodies in the late 1970s. And, even today, research continues in prestigious university research laboratories throughout the world.

Many authorities regard the different subtle bodies as 'octaves' of subtle energy or of consciousness within the same all-encompassing field.

## The mind, consciousness and beyond

Before going further it is worth considering the question of mind and consciousness a little further. Consciousness is essentially having an awareness of self as distinct from other beings and the environment. In the last chapter we fleetingly saw how Freud, Jung and Adler effectively transformed the discipline of psychiatry by postulating their very different theories of mind.

They all accepted the idea that the mind has two components, the conscious and the unconscious. Further, they accepted that the conscious was merely the tip of the iceberg, and as such could be studied. The unconscious, on the other hand, being 'submerged', so to speak, was open to conjecture. Their concepts about the unconscious led to their eventual split.

At this point suffice it to say that Freud believed that the unconscious was purely personal and that it was 'built' from developing experiences and childhood memories. Jung, however, went beyond this. He affirmed that man had a consciousness, and that beneath that there was a personal unconsciousness (although it was not furnished as was Freud's by sexualised developing experiences), but his concept went even deeper. He believed that beyond the personal unconscious there was a shared *collective unconscious*. This, he believed, was not inherited from one's forebears, but was in fact shared by all members of the human race, and was literally a universal consciousness. Here, we can see a distinct analogy with Sheldrake's Morphic Fields, and we can see how it could fit into Laszlo's psi-field (see Chapter One).

One could, of course, occupy several volumes in trying to define mind and its location — or non-location. The one thing that seems clear is that it seems to exist at several levels. In part, it is related to brain function, but also it seems to have no boundaries. If you focus on your mind itself for a while you will be aware it almost continually changes, fluctuates and shimmers. It is not so much a smoothly flowing process, but an ebbing and flowing field.

## Thought-field therapies

In recent years a growing number of surprisingly effective therapies have been developed to help people with various psychological problems, including phobias, anxiety and depression. They all are based on the concept of a thought field, which can be stimulated via one of the subtle energy systems in the individual.

In 1964 Dr George Goodheart, a chiropractor, discovered that certain muscle groups would become weak when opposing groups were in spasm. Stimulation of specific nodules associated with the weakened group seemed to cause an immediate improvement in the weakened group, simultaneously causing the spasm to go in the opposing group. Studying this phenomenon, and drawing on the work of an osteopath named Chapman, who had discovered certain organ reflexes, he devised a schema whereby he was able to diagnose and treat various organ malfunctions. Adding acupuncture to his study, Goodheart then discovered that certain meridians were also associated with the muscle groups on his schema. In 1974 he created a college for the study of his method, which was called Applied Kinesiology (AK).

One of Goodheart's students was clinical psychologist Dr Roger Callahan, who adapted the method to treat psychological problems. He found that by tapping on specific acupoints on specific meridians could eliminate some phobias in startlingly fast time. After lengthy research he devised the concept of *Thought-Field Therapy* (TFT) in about 1980.

Callahan's concept is that the thought field is a manifestation of the individual's energy system. Whenever one thinks, the thought field becomes active, or 'tuned in' to a particular thought. The body responds to this activity (possibly via PNI routes) for good or ill. Sometimes a *perturbation*, or blockage, will occur, so that whenever an individual has the particular thought associated with that perturbation, he will experience an inappropriate body response. For example, someone with agoraphobia may experience nausea, palpitations and increased perspiration (a panic attack) when simply thinking of going into a crowded environment.

In Thought-Field Therapy Dr Callahan developed an elaborate system for both diagnosing and treating problems using algorithms and various detailed sequences of tapping on specific meridian points. From it, a number of variants have developed, each of which has a slightly different emphasis.

Gary Craig, an electrical engineer and personal performance coach, trained under Dr Callahan and subsequently developed his method, called *Emotional Freedom Technique* (EFT). It is an altogether simpler approach, but seems to achieve excellent results.

Psychologist Francine Shapiro has devised *Eye Movement Desensitisation and Reprocessing* (EMDR) Therapy, which involves thinking about the problem area while moving the eyes back and forth in a particular manner, or being tapped at points on the body.

Yet another variant is *Matrix Work*, devised by Nahoma Clinton, which focuses on the chakras. In this, one works on core beliefs rather than feelings.

People able to see auras would aver that one can see the thought field, containing its thoughtforms and aberrations, which would correlate with Callahan's concept of perturbations.

So, let us move on and consider subtle anatomy.

## Subtle anatomy

George Engel, in a paper published in *Science* in 1976,[3] stated that a model is nothing more than a belief system utilised to explain natural phenomena, to make sense out of what is puzzling and disturbing.

In our discussion so far we have considered the various subtle bodies as a model of the different levels of being. We will now go a little further and consider three models by which the subtle bodies connect with the physical body.

### 1. THE CHAKRA AND NADI SYSTEM

This system is mentioned in both Hindu and Buddhist yogic literature, and in numerous esoteric texts. The *chakras* (from the Sanskrit word for 'wheel') are perceived as energy centres, or vortices, which penetrate the physical body and the subtle bodies, thereby linking the subtle fields. Each is associated with particular functions of the body, regulating the integrity and function of particular systems and organs, and different levels of consciousness. There are differences in the descriptions of these chakras in Hindu, Tibetan and Western texts, but this may be more to do with interpretation than actuality. As the late Osho described, 'some say that there are three, five, six, seven, eight or even nine major chakras. They are all correct!' Generally speaking, however, the commonest number given is seven.

The chakras are situated in a line along the spinal cord (Figure 4), each being associated with specific organs, functions, and particular endocrine glands. Thus:

*Base* — associated with large intestine and rectum, sharing responsibility for the kidneys. Also associated with the lower limbs and bone metabolism. Controls the adrenal glands. Governs excretory function. Generally associated with feelings of security,

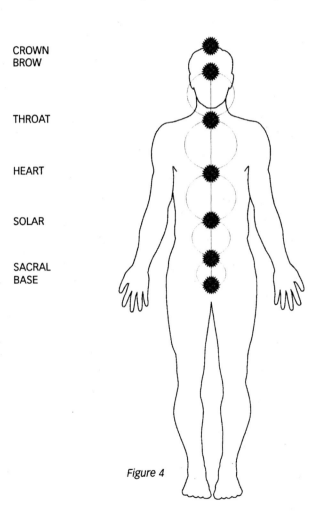

CROWN
BROW

THROAT

HEART

SOLAR

SACRAL
BASE

*Figure 4*

survival and grounding. Malfunctions may be associated with haemorrhoids, constipation, sciatica and obesity.

*Sacral* — associated with the uterus, ovaries, testicles, the bladder and sharing responsibility for the kidneys. Controls the endocrine function of the ovaries and the testicles. Governs reproductive function. Generally associated with emotions, sexuality, pleasure and creativity. Malfunctions may be associated with impotence, frigidity, both organic or functional sexual problems, bladder and kidney problems, emotional or psychological problems, back problems.

*Solar plexus* — associated with the liver, gall bladder, stomach, small intestine and spleen. Controls the endocrine function of the pancreas. Governs digestive function. Generally associated with will, power, drive, the 'fire in one's belly'. Malfunctions may be associated with ulcers, diabetes, hypoglycaemia, liver disease, eating disorders like anorexia and bulimia.

*Heart* — associated with the heart and the upper limbs, with shared responsibility for the lungs. Controls the function of the thymus. Governs the circulation. Generally associated with love of self and others, mental strength. Malfunctions may be associated with hypertension, heart disease, asthma and lung disease.

*Throat* — associated with the ears, neck, lungs and the throat, with shared responsibility for the lungs. Controls the function of the thyroid and parathyroid glands. Governs respiration and communicative functions. Generally associated with communication, self-expression, and creativity. Malfunctions may be associated with hearing difficulty, neck problems, thyroid disorders, and throat problems.

*Brow* — associated with the brain and eyes. Controls the function of the pituitary gland and pineal body. Governs cognition, vision, intuition and intellect. Generally associated with intuition, insight and perception. Malfunctions may be associated with headaches, visual problems, sleep disturbances and nightmares.

*Crown* — associated with the whole person. Controls the function of the hypothalamus, pineal body and pituitary gland. Governs higher intellectual functions, integration and understanding. Malfunctions may be associated with depression, alienation, and inability to comprehend or understand.

Each chakra can be in a state of balance, underactivity or overactivity. It can be blocked or unblocked. Malfunction can, therefore, have different profound effects upon the physical body.

But the chakras are not independent phenomena. They are linked in a network of channels, or *nadis* (from the Sanskrit for 'flow'), of which there are three main ones and literally thousands of minors. One text informs us that there are over 350,000 nadis in the body.

The main nadi, the *sushumna,* or central channel, arises from the base chakra and rises to the crown chakra. It has a balancing function.

The other two are the *ida* and the *pingala*. Ida is thought of as the moon, while pingala is thought of as the sun (i.e., they are polar energy flows). Ida emerges from the right of the base chakra, weaving in and out between the chakras, while pingala emerges from the left and also weaves its way in and out, until they meet with sushumna at the brow chakra, before continuing as a single current.

## 2. THE MERIDIAN SYSTEM

Fundamental to Traditional Chinese Medicine is the concept that Qi (pronounced Ch'i), the universal primal energy, flows through the body in an ordered sequence along specific pathways called *meridians* (Figure 5). Originally these were thought to be channels like arteries and veins, but no such anatomical structures have

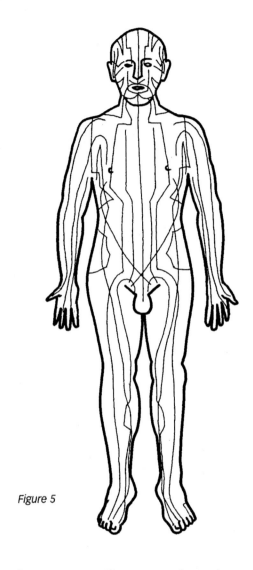

*Figure 5*

ever been shown to exist. There are twelve main meridians, each of which is related to a particular organ. They are bilateral; twelve on each side of the body, on each of which there are a series of *acupoints*. In addition, there are two central meridians, one on the front of the body and one on the back.

Originally, 365 acupoints were described, in keeping with the all-important system of numbers in Chinese philosophy, but this number has since been extended to over a thousand. It is important to realise, however, that the points are not merely surface points as is implied by the acupuncture maps, but are effective at varying depths below the skin. The maps can, therefore, best be thought of like maps of underground train systems.

It is appropriate to mention at this point *Qigong* (pronounced Ch'i gong). This literally means 'work on the Qi'. Practitioners of Qigong use mind control to move and control the Qi in order to improve health and maintain balance and harmony. They effectively work on the body's energy field.

As mentioned above, Qi is thought in Traditional Chinese Medicine to flow through all living things and the environment. In the body it flows along the meridians, exchanging at acupoints with the Qi in the environment. Thus, the body's field is in connection with the environment and with the energy fields of all living things.

### 3. THE DIRECT ETHERIC-PHYSICAL INTERFACE

The etheric body is considered by many people to be virtually an energetic double of the physical body, akin to the Ka of the ancient Egyptians. In this model every tissue, organ and system of the physical body is conceived as having its counterpart in the etheric. The two are seen as being in direct dynamic association, so that imbalance in the etheric kidney, for example, would have a manifestation in the physical kidney. However, whereas the physical body can become substantially altered by pathological processes, trauma, or the removal of organs and limbs by surgery, the etheric body maintains its integrity. Removal of an organ, for example, does not result in removal of the etheric organ, but is merely reflected in an alteration in the functional control which the etheric body holds over the physical.

Note that the term model is still used in the context of the direct etheric-physical interface, since modern thinking considers the etheric body to be more likely to be a field than an etheric mirror image. As such it seems to be holographic, every point in the field containing information about the totality of the physical body.

These three subtle systems can be thought of as transducing systems between the etheric and higher subtle bodies and the physical body. They are different, have different functions, yet undoubtedly also have many overlaps. And, indeed, if we consider them all as being part of a unifying field their roles and their overlaps become so much more understandable.

It is also worth mentioning the Unitary Theory of Disease, and the role of protein, which will be discussed more fully in Chapter Seven. Dr George Laurence believed that this explained much about the connection between the etheric and the physical levels.

## The psi-field

We are now going to construct a model of the psi-field to illustrate just how all of the elements that we have considered in this chapter come together. But before we do so, we shall return to an analogy from ancient Egypt. As we do so, however, please understand that the reason for using Egyptian symbolism is simply because they as a people thought in terms of symbols as they tried to fathom the nature of life in relation to Nature. And some of their symbolism was, in fact, extremely apposite.

Everyone is aware that the ancient Egyptian pantheon was huge. They saw divinity in everything and symbolised virtually every activity by the worship of a god or goddess, generally represented as a human form with the head of an animal or other creature. The eighteenth dynasty pharaoh, Amunhotep IV, shortly after he ascended to the throne, changed all that. Sweeping aside all of the old gods he decreed that there should be only one god worshipped throughout Egypt. This was the Aten, or the sun disk. To show his devotion he renamed himself *Akenaten*, literally 'the spirit of Aten'.[4]

During Akenaten's reign, often referred to as the *Amarna Period*, because the pharaoh moved his capital, his city of dreams, to a new location in the desert, there was a short-lived renaissance in the arts. In depictions of people the portrayal of the Aten became symbolic of Akenaten's belief that life was given directly by the god. The Aten, the sun disk, is shown with sunbeams ending in hands. Wherever they touch a human, there is a hand holding an ankh, the symbol of life, to the face of the subject (Figure 6).

Akenaten believed that all life was sacred and that blood should no longer be spilled in sacrifices. His depiction of the life force coming straight from the source of his universe is a symbol of great profundity.

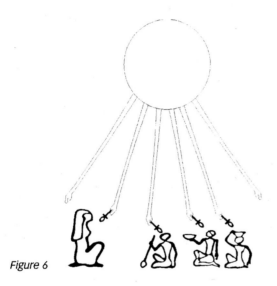

Figure 6

It is also a model that we can adapt further in our journey to interpret the psi-field. Understand that, for simplicity, this is a three-dimensional model.

By virtue of three dimensionality we have a starting point, which is convenient, because it is conceptualised as the source.[5] From this source, like a sun, an infinite number of beams radiate in every direction.[6] The tip of each beam represents a 'thing' in the universe, from a subatomic particle to a galaxy, from a unicellular organism to a human being. In their own beam they are unique from every other, yet they are all connected to the unifying source.

We are mainly concerned here with humankind, so from now we consider the beam spreading out from the source as being a person. This individual has an essence, which we call soul. This is connected *with* the unifying source, yet has individuality.

The beam passes through several influencing fields (Figure 7), the deepest being the *collective unconscious*, followed by a *morphogenetic field*, then possibly by a *karmic field* and a *field of acquisition*. Thus the soul, the individual's essence is connected to the collective unconscious, giving access to universal thoughtforms

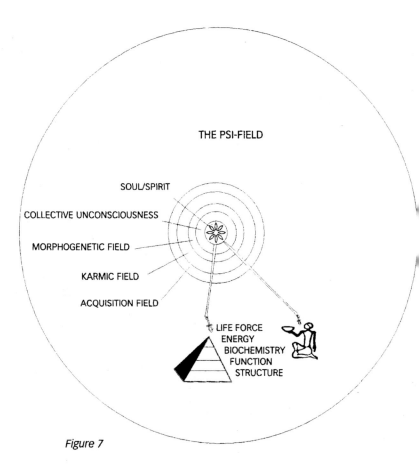

THE PSI-FIELD

SOUL/SPIRIT

COLLECTIVE UNCONSCIOUSNESS

MORPHOGENETIC FIELD

KARMIC FIELD

ACQUISITION FIELD

LIFE FORCE
ENERGY
BIOCHEMISTRY
FUNCTION
STRUCTURE

*Figure 7*

and archetypal memories, and is then subject to species memory and formative forces (encompassing both Sheldrake's concept and Steiner's ideas about formative forces). Karmic and acquisition fields would seem to be more specific, relating to smaller numbers of individuals (in this model, small clusters of beams) so that forebears and other influences upon the individual can have a direct input into the individual's life. These influences can be partly genetic and partly acquired energetically.

In the illustration we have retained the ancient Egyptian symbol of the *ankh*, the life principle, because it is precisely that, a good symbol for the vital energy which we know as life.

And the hand and ankh touch the pyramid of life, which like the sun rays touching the pyramids of Egypt symbolises the connection between the energetic and the physical.

This then is the psi-field, a holographic information system containing the entire history of the universe, every thought, action, interaction, birth, life and death. It is everywhere and nowhere at the same time, for it underlies the vacuum in all space.

## The personal psi-field

The beam of light is one's life. It is the individual; it is unique to that individual and it too has many facets. It has been subject to the fields that we have discussed, which are responsible for forming us, for good or ill, into the unique people we are.

We can think of the beam touching our personal pyramid (of life as well as the pyramid of medicine), and that energetic capstone interconnects with, controls and maintains the physical body. One can think of the beam of light as being the personal psi-field, and the capstone as being the etheric body (which is also a part of the psi-field, as is the body) containing:

- Thought field — containing the emotions and mind
- Chakric system
- Meridian system
- The direct etheric–physical interface

This is the vitalising part of the individual. It is far more subtle than electromagnetic impulses and chemical reactions, although they are the result, the manifestation of the interaction of the energetic field with the physical body.

And one can also see how the pyramid of medicine, which doctors have been busily building over the eons, begins to make sense. Psychoneuroimmunology begins to make sense. Thought field therapies begin to make sense. Acupuncture and all sorts of therapies begin to make sense, because anything which is done at the physical level must have an effect on the individual's psi-field, which brings into play the individual's self-regulating mechanisms.

This is of course precisely what Hippocrates and others have meant when they have talked about the healing power of nature — *Vis Medicatrix Naturae*. It is the 'body' (that is, the mind, body and spirit, not just the physical body) which is continually trying its hardest to make the best of a bad job. Whatever the body has, whatever it has thrown at it, the 'body' will do the best that it can. Often it protests — produces symptoms, which are perceived as illness — but it does the best that it can. The role of the physician is to allow it to do so in the best manner possible.

### Interconnectedness

It is appropriate here to talk again about this phenomenon, since it is at the very heart of Psionic Medicine.

People are often confused as to how one can tell anything about an individual by analysing a sample that was removed from the body some time previously (indeed, possibly years before). After all, logic would normally dictate that the only information that one could elicit would relate to the chemical state of affairs in the specimen from the static point in time when the sample was removed from the body. Well, that would be true if one were merely analysing it chemically. But in psionic analysis we are not doing that. We are analysing the specimen energetically, by tuning into the personal psi-field of which it is a part. And because we are tuning into the psi-field, the information that is obtainable is current in that it tells us about the state of energies that are operational and that are affecting the individual at that very moment in time.

In Chapter One we discussed the concept of interconnectedness at the quantum level. This is reality not some abstruse hypothetical interpretation of the universe. The truth is that we live in an interconnected universe, which seems to have holographic features. And in our discussion in this chapter we have looked at the psi-field and have tried to explain it and our place within it through the use of models.

In Psionic Medicine we use a sample of the patient's protein, be that a blood sample or a lock of hair, to tune into their personal psi-field, as well as into the total psi-field. Essentially, all of the matter that has ever been part of the physical body of the individual is made up of molecules, atoms and particles. All of those particles have interacted,[7] so that even when they are separated they continue to interact through *non-local* connections. The specimen furnishes a means of discovering what is currently taking place within the personal psi-field of the patient. This means that one can tap into the information about that individual in their psi-field, because the specimen is and always will be a part of that personal psi-field.

## A new view

Man, being a rational being, is constantly striving to understand his universe and his place within it. In order to get on with our daily life it seems important to have a frame of reference, a basis upon which we can make sense of what happens to us and the world around us. The development of a belief system of some sort helps us to do this. Indeed, it is almost innate. To the scientist the belief may be in science, to the theologian (and in this context, one means any follower of any religion) it is a belief in spirit, and to the atheist it is belief in non-belief.

Sir James Frazer (1854–1941), regarded as the founder of

modern anthropology, wrote in his book, *The Golden Bough*, that evolving societies move through a process of development which involves the three phases of magic, religion and science. Living in the scientific age as we do, it is easy to look back at earlier civilisations and societies and smile at the naivety of their beliefs. This presupposes that this progression through the phases is advancement, that the scientific view is better than the religious or spiritual, or that the spiritual is better than the so-called magic or mystical. It is another presupposition to say that they are even mutually exclusive.

The concept of an all-pervasive holographic information system, the psi-field, is a new and quite mind-boggling concept. It can be viewed from any of the phases one wishes and be understandable. It does not demand that one takes a particular view, but it accords with all views.

Indeed, as Ervin Laszlo says in his book, *The Whispering Pond*, 'the emerging insight is not a throwback to previous, now outdated concepts.' He concludes, 'the current shift in science's concept of the world from a lifeless rock to an interconnected and quasi-living universe has intense meaning and significance for our times. The concept of a subtly interconnected world, of a whispering pond in and through which we are intimately linked to each other and to the universe, assimilated by our intellect and embraced by our heart, is part of humanity's response to the challenges that we now face in common. Our separation from each other and from nature is at the root of many of our problems; overcoming them calls for a recovery of our neglected, but never entirely forgotten, bonds and connections.'

We will consider how distortions of the personal psi-field can result in illness when we come to consider the psionic method in Chapter Eleven.

---

[1] The Akashic Records are a theosophical concept. The word comes from the Sanskrit *akasha*, defined as the ether or all-pervasive space. It can be seen that this could easily be viewed as the psi-field.

[2]Sir Oliver Lodge was professor of Physics at Liverpool University, and a man who influenced the early career of George Laurence.

[3]See footnote, Chapter Three.

[4]Akenaten, the so-called 'heretic pharaoh' ascended the throne of Egypt in about 1377 BC and ruled for 16 years. With his wife Nefertiti ('the beautiful one cometh') he tried to establish monotheism. He was described by J.H. Breasted, (from his chapter in the first edition of *The Cambridge Ancient History*) as 'the first individual in history'.

[5]If we conceptualise this as a holographic effect then all points are one; thus the source is not restricted to a specific location, but exists throughout the holographic field.

[6]An alternative model is to think of a fibre-optic lamp, the fibres forming a sphere, each fibre producing its own unique pinpoint of light.

[7]See Bell's Theorem in Chapter One.

# Homoeopathy — The Subtle Medicine

*'Similia similibus curentur.'*
(Let like be treated by like.)

**Samuel Hahnemann**

omoeopathy is a gentle form of medicine which was known to the ancient Greeks, a fact mirrored by its derivation from the Greek *homoios*, meaning 'like', and *pathos*, meaning 'suffering'. Essentially, it means treating like with like.

It was the great Hippocrates who first taught that there are two ways of treating a patient: one could either treat with 'contraries', or with 'similarities'. That is, one could either give medication to counteract symptoms — the *law of contraries* — or give medication which had the ability to produce the same symptoms as those experienced or suffered by the person — the *law of similars*. In both cases he believed that the physician was merely creating the right conditions for the inner healing power, *Vis Medicatrix Naturae*, to bring about a cure.

Several hundred years later in sixteenth-century Europe, Theophrastis Bombastus von Hohenheim, otherwise known as Paracelsus (1493–1541), threw off the shackles of medical dogmatism and again taught the merits of treating like with like. It was not, however, until the eighteenth century that the basic principles became formalised into a true system of medicine.

## Dr Samuel Hahnemann (1755–1843)

The founder of this system of medicine was an eccentric genius by the name of Samuel Christian Hahnemann, the son of a china-painter in the famous Meissen pottery works. After qualifying in Medicine from the University of Erlangen in 1779, he practised for several years before becoming disenchanted with the rather brutal and dubious medical treatments of the day. As a result he gave up medical practice, started studying chemistry, and eked out a modest living by writing and translating.

In 1790, while translating a textbook written by the famous Scottish physician William Cullen (1712–1790) (the professor of both Medicine and Chemistry at Edinburgh University, and one of the founders of the school of medicine at Glasgow University), Hahnemann came across a section dealing with the treatment of malaria with quinine. Although this was (and still is) an appropriate treatment for the disease, he was unconvinced by Cullen's explanation that it worked by virtue of having a tonic effect upon the stomach. He reasoned that, since other more powerful 'tonics' had no such beneficial effect, it had to be working by some other mechanism. Accordingly, experimentalist that he was, he dosed himself with quinine for several days, the result being that he began to experience the symptoms of malaria.

Thus the germ of an idea began to form — a drug that produced the symptoms of an illness in a healthy subject could also be used to treat an illness with the same characteristics.

Over the following years Hahnemann returned to medical practice, developing the concept of *similia similibus curentur*, by dosing himself, his family and friends with different substances in order to study the symptoms produced when they were given to healthy subjects. These experiments came to be known as *provings*, from the German word *prufung*, meaning 'testing'. In 1796 he produced an article entitled *An Essay on a new principle for ascertaining the curative power of drugs*. This was the first of a series of articles in which his developing ideas become apparent. Then in 1806 he published *The Medicine of Experience*, a work that gives us our first clear glimpse of the system he was working on. Indeed, a year later in 1807 he first used the term 'Homoeopathy'.

Further work culminated in the publication in 1810 of his book *Organon of Rational Healing*. In it, in aphorism style, he set down his developing ideas for his system of homoeopathic medicine. The choice of title is interesting, because it comes from the Greek, *Organum*, meaning 'tool'. Two possible reasons why he chose the word come from two thinkers and their method of writing. First was Aristotle, whose various treatises on logic were summed up under the common title *Organon*. The other was Bacon, whose method of inductive reasoning was outlined in his book *Novum Organon*. Indeed, Hahnemann's use of aphorisms is very much in keeping with the layout of Bacon's *Novum Organum*.

The *Organon of Medicine* (Hahnemann changed the title in the second edition) went through five editions and modifications during his lifetime, the last being published in 1833, although the manuscript for a sixth edition was completed before he died in 1843.[1] This fifth edition contained additional material on Hahnemann's concepts of the Vital Force and, highly relevant to homoeopathy today, what he called the 'dynamization of medicines'.

Initially, Hahnemann had prescribed his remedies in the standard doses of the day. However, although his results were good, he found that many of his patients suffered an initial aggravation of their symptoms before receiving the benefit. In an attempt to counter this he started giving one-tenth doses. The results were still good, but the aggravations, though less marked, still occurred. He therefore continued diluting the doses, each time giving a tenth of the previous dose. Predictably, the aggravations disappeared, but so too did any beneficial effect. The dilutions had reached a point where there was no more medication present.

Homoeopathy might have died a death at that point had Hahnemann not discovered an incredible phenomenon. He found that by vigorously shaking each progressive dilution, the resultant remedy became not only less likely to produce aggravations, but it became more potent. This process he called *Dynamization*. Today, we call it *Potentisation*.

Fundamental to his theory of homoeopathy by this stage was the concept of the Vital Force. It was his view that the remedy acted not upon the disease but upon the Vital Force to restore balance within the body.

Between 1812 and 1821, while he was Professor of Medicine at Leipzig, Hahnemann published a six-volume work entitled The *Materia Medica Pura*. It contained the results of all his provings. However, because of a legal wrangle with the apothecaries who tried to sue him on the grounds that he was infringing their right to prepare drugs, he was forced to leave the city and move to Köthen. It was there that he wrote a five-volume work entitled *The Chronic Diseases*. This, together with the *Organon* and the *Materia Medica Pura* formed the basic texts of his homoeopathic theory.

In *The Chronic Diseases*, Hahnemann set out to explain why homoeopathy sometimes worked well with acute illnesses, yet failed with chronic disease. He postulated that chronic diseases were due to one of three miasms, which he termed *Psora, Sycosis and Syphilis*. He believed that they were disturbances in the Vital Force which permeates the body. Sometimes these miasms, from the Greek *miainein*, meaning 'stain or pollute', could be acquired and sometimes they were inherited, thereby exerting an effect through several generations, like 'ghosts of the original illness'.

Hahnemann believed that the *psoric group*, which related to *'suppressed itch'* from the all-too-common scabies, accounted for about 75 per cent of all chronic ailments, especially congestive states, skin and spinal disorders and tuberculosis. It was also associated with extreme restlessness, fears and oversensitiveness.

The other two groups he thought accounted for the remainder of chronic conditions, in about equal measures. The *sycotic group*, derived from a gonorrhoeal origin, he associated with warts, growths, catarrh and rheumatic problems. The syphilitic group, derived from syphilis, seemed to relate to cardiac, neurological and degenerative conditions including a tendency to ulceration.

## The spread of homoeopathy

By the time of Hahnemann's death at the age of 88 in 1843, homoeopathy had spread far and wide. In England, Dr Harvey Quin founded the British Homoeopathic Society in 1844 and was instrumental in opening the London Homoeopathic Hospital in 1850.

Other converts to the method carried it further afield. By the end of the nineteenth century there were homoeopathic hospitals all over Europe, Russia, the two Americas and the Indian subcontinent.

## Dr James Tyler Kent (1849–1916)

In the USA, sometime in the mid 1870s, a young orthodox-trained physician by the name of James T. Kent called upon the services of a homoeopathic doctor to tend to his ill wife. Standard orthodox treatment had failed to help her so she had begged him to try the new medicine. To Kent's surprise a dramatic cure was achieved. From then on Dr Kent determined to find out more about this amazing method. It proved to be a fortunate day for the development of homoeopathy.

Hahnemann and his followers had proved around 130 remedies, but over the few years since his death the number had swollen considerably. However, although the body of knowledge had grown, it remained fairly disorganised. That is where Kent proved his worth. He systematised the materia medica to give a clearer picture of each remedy. His work, published in three major volumes: *Lectures on Homoeopathic Philosophy*; *Lectures on Homoeopathic Materia Medica*, and *The Repertory of the Homoeopathic Materia Medica*, became the foundation for homoeopathic training for decades to come. Indeed, 'Kent's Repertory', as his last work is known around the world, is probably still the single most commonly used tool for homoeopaths today. Essentially, it is a book containing every conceivable symptom and the manner in which it is perceived by the individual, or modified by external agents such as temperature, weather, movement, etc. It is organised into logical sections and is cross-indexed against all of the appropriate remedies.

## Dr Edward Bach (1886–1936)

Many people around the world know the name of Edward Bach, since he was the originator of the wonderful system of treatment which bears his name — the Bach Flower Remedies. He was an orthodox-trained doctor who had specialised in bacteriology and homoeopathy.

In the 1920s Dr Edward Bach practised as a pathologist at the London Homoeopathic Hospital and as a homoeopathic physician in Harley Street. In that time he produced a stream of scientific papers and worked with Dr John Paterson in the development of the bowel nosodes, an important group of remedies.[2] For this work he was acclaimed by his colleagues as 'the second Hahnemann'.

Bach's real aim in life was to produce the simplest form of medicine possible, which could be taken by the sufferer him or herself without fear or harm. In 1930, having become disillusioned with the scientific method (much to do with his creative and intuitive nature) he threw up his practice and moved to the country.

He thought that certain negative states of mind resulted in illness, and that by correcting the emotional imbalances a whole-person cure could be obtained. He sought and found these remedies among the flowers of the fields and hedgerows of the English countryside.

Initially, he found 12 plants which were capable of correcting 12 corresponding negative states of mind. His findings were duly written up in his book *Heal Thyself* and the world famous *The Twelve Healers*. In the years between 1933 and his death in 1936 he found another 26 remedies to complete the 38 remedies which seem to cover most of the negative states of mind that are commonly suffered from.

## The Principles of Homoeopathy

From the preceding brief historical outline it should be fairly clear that the two main principles are the Law of Similars and the use of potentised remedies. Let us now look at them in a little more detail.

### THE LAW OF SIMILARS

This means that a substance, which produces symptoms of a disease in a well person, can also be used to treat someone who has that disease. Hence, *similia similibus curentur* – let like be treated by like.

Effectively one takes the symptom-complex of the patient and attempts to match it up with the toxic effect-complex of a remedy. There may be several remedies which are close, but the nearest match is the *similar*. As an example, belladonna poisoning causes a toxic effect-complex, which resembles the disease of scarlet fever. If someone suffering with a scarlet-fever-like illness presents in the classic manner, then belladonna would be the appropriate similar.

This is a fairly clear-cut case. It is important to appreciate, however, that in homoeopathy one is trying to match the remedy profile to the patient profile, not simply to the disease profile. To explain this, consider five men all of whom have arthritis affecting their hips. The same orthodox treatment may be appropriate for all five. A homoeopath, however, would look at the symptom patterns of each individual and could well end up prescribing a completely different remedy for each man. It is, after all, the individual that is being treated in homoeopathy and not the disease.

### POTENCY AND THE INFINITESIMAL DOSE

Although homoeopathy is associated with using infinitesimal amounts of substances, it is the Law of Similars which is the crux of the method. If the incorrect remedy is chosen, the question of potency is almost irrelevant.

The modern homoeopathic materia medica contains well over two thousand remedies. All sorts of things are used, from simple substances like common salt, to exotic cacti, snake venoms and precious elements like gold. They can all be prepared in different potencies.

Potency means far more than dilution. The process of potentisation actually seems to enhance the 'power' of the remedy, so that it becomes more potent. The remedy becomes less concentrated but more energised.

In order to prepare homoeopathic remedies two standard methods are used (although there are other methods). Firstly, for soluble substances an alcoholic extract is made by infusion for up to three weeks, followed by filtration to produce a *mother tincture* (commonly indicated by the symbol $\phi$). This is then diluted with 40 per cent alcohol to 1:10 or 1:100. Next it is vigorously vibrated for a few seconds, a process called *succussion*, to produce the first potency remedy on the two commonest potency scales. The 1:10 scale is called the *Decimal scale* (which was first introduced by Dr Constantine Hering — see endnote[5]) and is designated by the letter 'x' in the UK, and by 'D' on the continent. Thus the first potency on the Decimal scale would be 1x.

The 1:100 scale is called the *Centesimal scale* (which was Hahnemann's original potency scale) and is designated by the letter 'c' in the UK, and by 'CH' on the continent. The first potency on the Centesimal scale would be 1c.

To prepare the next potency one part of the first potency would be taken and diluted 1:10 or 1:100, then succussed as before to produce the 2x or 2c potencies.

It will now be very clear that it does not take many dilutions to dramatically reduce the concentration of a substance. By the sixth process on the Decimal scale, which is the equivalent of the third on the Centesimal scale (in concentration, but not in energetic terms) the mother tincture will be diluted to one in a million, or $10^{-6}$. By the sixth process on the Centesimal scale the dilution will be one in a billion. These figures are quite incredible. Indeed, by the time one reaches the 12c potency, applying *Avogadro's hypothesis*,[3] it is unlikely that there will be a single molecule left of the original substance.

The second method is for insoluble substances, which cannot be made into mother tinctures. In this case they are mechanically ground together with lactose powder for several hours in the proportion of 1:10 or 1:100 (depending upon which potency scale is used), a process called *trituration*. This process is repeated to the 6x or the 3c level (which are both the equivalent of 1:1,000,000 or $10^{-6}$ ) after which it can be dissolved in alcohol and water and potentised in the usual manner.

By convention 12c is the cut off point, all remedies up to this being considered low potency and those of 12c and above being high potency. Remedies are prepared up to inordinate potencies, the *Millesimals* (equivalent to a thousand c), designated 'M'. Hence, 1M (1,000c), 10M (10,000c), 50M (50,000c) and CM (100,000c).

There is another scale called the *LM scale* (the 50,000 scale), which is actually a composite method of producing potentised remedies.[4] It is achieved by trituration with lactose to the 3c level, which is the starting point. Thereafter, serial dilutions of 1:50,000 are made in liquid, with one hundred succussions at each stage, producing LM1, LM2, LM3 and so on. Advocates of the LM scale claim fewer aggravations than with other potency scales.

### THE LAW OF CURE

Another of the main homoeopathic principles is the Law of Cure, formulated by an American homoeopath, Constantine Hering[5] (Figure 8). It states that a cure is effected:

- From above downwards
- From within outwards
- From major to lesser organs
- In reverse order of the appearance of the symptoms

HERING'S LAW OF CURE

1) FROM ABOVE DOWN

2) FROM WITHIN OUT

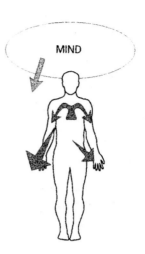

3) FROM MAJOR TO LESSER ORGANS

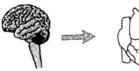   

4) IN REVERSE ORDER OF SYMPTOMS

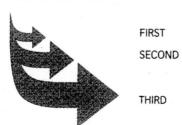

FIRST

SECOND

THIRD

*Figure 8*

## THE CURRENT STATE OF HOMOEOPATHY

Within the world of homoeopathy today there are many different schools of thought. Although they all fundamentally adhere to the basic ideas first promulgated by Samuel Hahnemann there are broadly diverging opinions as to whether a single remedy (classical homoeopathy) or multiple remedies (pluralistic homoeopathy) should be given; whether to prescribe according to miasms (miasmatic prescribing), constitutional types (constitutional prescribing), or pathological conditions (local or pathological prescribing).

Constitutional prescribing is by and large used in Greece and India, whereas local prescribing is favoured in France and Latin America. In the UK there is generally a mix of the two, constitutional remedies being used to boost the immune system and pathological or local remedies being used to deal with the symptoms of the illness.

Similarly, there are differing opinions about which potencies should be used, either high or low. This, of course, has been a problem every since the introduction of homoeopathy. Hahnemann himself advocated using the 30c, while Kent would never use lower than 30c. Indeed, he often used far higher potencies, even going up to the millionth (MM) on the Centesimal scale.

Again, there is no conformity of opinion worldwide as to which potency is used. Indeed, most homoeopaths would be happy if the whole question of potency simply disappeared. For this reason many people restrict themselves to the use of perhaps three or four potencies, the selection of which is entirely decided by rule of thumb.

## PSIONIC MEDICINE ADDS A NEW DIMENSION

Homoeopathy is not an easy discipline to practise, because it takes a long time to learn the materia medica, and to get into the habit of taking a good case history in order to build up a picture of the patient and his or her experience of life. And it is understanding their experience which is so important. By going into the minutiae of their symptoms, eliciting the way they react, think, and express themselves, all this and much more, allows the skilled homoeopath to produce a patient-profile. This then has to be matched as closely as possible with an appropriate remedy-profile. The closer the match, the better the result.

As mentioned above, there are different approaches used throughout the world. Some homoeopaths, for example, may always prescribe constitutionally, while others may go straight for the pathological remedy. At times the choice will seem clear, while at other times it may be a matter of going for whichever seems to best come out of the questioning.

Psionic Medicine techniques add an extra dimension to both remedy selection and potency choice, by finding out in a precise manner. Effectively, it is as if they provide a laboratory and X-ray facility to transform homoeopathy from an art into a science.

There are very often several approaches which will help some-one at any one time. There will, however, be a hierarchical order in which it is best to do so. A psionic approach will indicate the best one, which may not be so apparent to the classical homoeopath.

And on the potency question, while many classical homoeopaths would say that the potency is not really all that important (the correct remedy being essential), psionic experience indicates that the correct potency is vital. Indeed, not only is the potency level vital in terms of treatment, but it is important in terms of making the diagnosis of the cause of the patient's problem. This may con-fuse a lot of homoeopaths, but this is simply because a traditional question and answer approach to homoeopathy is not adequate in order to open up the avenues which have to be searched.

This is something that we shall reconsider in Chapter Eleven, when we come to examine the psionic approach.

### AND FINALLY, A WORD FROM DR GEORGE LAURENCE

Let us see what Dr George Laurence himself had to say upon this subject:[6]

*'While in most respects homoeopathic medicines are more efficient and certainly much safer than the orthodox, and that by using the*

principle of "similia similibus curentur" I admit that spectacular results are often obtained — I presume by removing the underlying cause of the aberration of the protein, as McDonagh[7] would have it. But there always seems to be too much of trial and error in the system and a lack of consistency in the approach of its practitioners.

'I know that, like the orthodox, we can dodge the issue by calling our practice an art, but I feel that we should do better and make such progress as would justify us in calling it a science. And that, I am convinced, can only be done by studying and making use of the psionic method, which has now been proved to be of inestimable value.

'Again in reading the homoeopathic journals, both our own and the American, one cannot help being struck by the long lists of remedies which have been tried in a given case before a satisfactory result could be obtained.

'Can we remain complacent with that?

'I am afraid that I have stressed these points but I feel that they need emphasising and facing up to. It is no good homoeopaths just sitting down and thinking that what Hahnemann said was the truth, the whole truth and nothing but the truth, when actually that portentous thinker would have been the very first to have welcomed any advance which would have proved his unique theories, or otherwise have promoted the cause of homoeopathy.

'If the psionic approach does nothing else, it proves Hahnemann's hypothesis of the miasms beyond a shadow of a doubt.'

### – AND HIS VIEW ON POTENCY

'It is little short of amazing how, with a little practice, the pendulum will pick out the appropriate remedy, and moreover tell you quite definitely which potency is likely to be the most effective. This is of special value, as in orthodox homoeopathic teaching the question of potencies is always a stumbling block and depends very much on the personal preference or experience of the practitioner. Furthermore, the pendulum can give you a very good idea of the exact dosage and the length of time for which the remedy should be prescribed.'

[1]The sixth edition of *Organon of Medicine* was published in 1921.

[2]See Chapter Six.

[3]*Amedeo Avogadro*, Conte di Quaregna, 1776–1856, was an Italian physicist. In 1811 he proposed his famous hypothesis which allowed scientists to calculate the Avogadro Number, the number of molecules in a gram-molecule.

[4]Hahnemann used first the Centesimal scale, and later introduced the 50,000 scale. For interest, see the Organon, para 270 (which was wholly rewritten for the sixth edition) and its appropriate footnotes.

[5]Dr Constantine Hering, (1800–1880), often called the Father of Homoeopathy in America, graduated MD from the University of Würzburg. He arrived in Philadelphia, USA in 1833 and established a Homoeopathic School at Allentown, Pennsylvania, which came to be known as the Allentown Academy. He researched and wrote widely, proving 72 drugs, including Cantharis, Psorinum, Lachesis, Nux moschata and Gelsemium. He is famous for his Law of Cure, and for introducing the Decimal scale of potency.

[6]Taken from a paper on Psionic Medicine, read to the Medical Society for the Study of Radiesthesia, London 1962.

[7]See Chapter Seven on The Unitary Theory of Disease.

# Miasms and Toxins

Dr Farley Spink
Dean of the Institute of Psionic Medicine

## 1

### Hahnemann's three miasms

The concept of *miasms,* or deep-seated morbid processes under-lying the common manifestations of illness, has always been central to the theory and practice of Psionic Medicine, as also of the Classical homoeopathic approach to the treatment of chronic disease. First proposed by Hahnemann,[1] nearly two hundred years ago, it attempted to explain his observations that acute ail-ments, even when successfully treated with homoeopathy, never-theless often recurred. He was, however, drastically handicapped by the total lack at the time of any of our modern laboratory and other diagnostic facilities, and indeed by the still very sketchy understanding of the mechanisms of disease. Consequently he was able only to trace a definite link between the two well-known venereal diseases, Syphilis and Gonorrhoea, and manifestations occurring later in the same patient or, more importantly, in their descendants.

He considered that these antecedent causes accounted for about 10 per cent of the problems he was called upon to treat. The remaining 90 per cent he was forced to include in a single vast category attributed to the third miasm which he called Psora, and which he associated with the consequences of external treatment and resulting suppression of skin disorders. But he still regarded it, like the others, as *contagious*, although we now know that the majority of skin diseases are nothing of the kind. Relatively primitive though his theory was, it was nevertheless a brilliant and basic concept, which enabled him to make great advances in the efficiency of homoeopathic methods. His book *Chronic Diseases* elaborates at great length on his thinking, and describes a large number of new remedies to deal with the three miasmatic states and their manifestations.

Unfortunately, because the idea, as propounded by Hahnemann, is so patently, in our modern eyes, merely a beginning, the germ only, of a real understanding of the nature of disease, it has given rise to two equally irrational attitudes in recent times. There are many homoeopaths who take the view that the original thesis cannot be improved upon — *'the gospel according to Hahnemann'*, if you like.[2] There are also others who, by reason of its obvious incompleteness, dismiss the whole thing as nonsense. To try to present a rational update of this most valuable concept is the object of this chapter.

Despite the foregoing remarks, it is striking that the described characteristics of the original *'three'* nonetheless do correspond with the three fundamental types of manifestations of disease, namely: overproliferation of tissue (*Sycosis — gonorrhoeal miasm*); destruction and ulceration (*Syphilitic*); and functional depletion and imbalance (*Psora*). And, regarded in this light, the theory is indeed a monument to Hahnemann's genius and acuteness of observation.

## THE TUBERCULOSIS MIASM

The advent of modern technology, beginning, so far as medicine is concerned, with Pasteur's work on bacteria in the mid-nineteenth century (some twenty years after Hahnemann's death) and leading on to the discovery of viruses, together with the development of biochemistry and endocrinology, opened up new knowledge which could be applied by homoeopaths as well as conventional doctors. Of particular importance was the discovery by Robert Koch, published in 1882, of the causal organism of tuberculosis. The *nosodes* (homoeopathic potentised preparations of disease products) of gonorrhoea and syphilis had been introduced some years before this, and Hahnemann himself used *Psorinum* (made from the 'itch pustule' — the exact nature being uncertain). But, hard on the heels of Koch, James Compton Burnett,[2] a famous homoeopathic physician in London, published his book on the uses of *Bacillinum*, made from tuberculous tissue, and described many features of what we now call the TB miasm, clearly recognisable in later generations who have never been in contact with the disease.

So important is this as a major underlying cause of chronic ailments that it has to be given rank alongside the two great 'infective' miasms of Hahnemann. In fact there would seem to be an evolutionary 'stacking order': *Syphilis* being probably the most ancient and deepest, its manifestations often not surfacing until old age; next *TB*, showing up at all ages, but responsible for a host of, for examples, arthritic, endocrine, chest and probably allergic disorders; lastly *Sycosis*, 'the miasm of our time', also with a great range of effects, particularly of a catarrhal nature, and going on to heart disease and cancer, the ultimate products of the whole miasmatic process.

George Laurence[3] established, very early in his work on Psionic Medicine, the overwhelming importance of the TB miasm.

### THE ACQUIRED TOXINS

It also soon became apparent that the various virus diseases can leave damaging 'hangovers', which often have to be eradicated before the major miasms can be dealt with. These factors have been called *'acquired toxins'* (to distinguish them from 'inherited miasms') and in at least some instances are due to persistence of the actual infective agent in the organism, for example the chickenpox virus, which can resurface years later as shingles. The distinction is somewhat blurred, however, since by psionic methods, a hangover of measles, for example, and very often of smallpox vaccination, can be picked up in patients who have never themselves been exposed to the relevant infection. An interesting item that seems to have been completely overlooked is smallpox itself, a mass killer in the past, but increasingly rare during the twentieth century and extinct now since 1979. It nevertheless shows up on Psionic analysis in many people and may prove to be important.

Many of the viruses seem to have a definite relationship with one or other of the major miasms, for example: measles, influenza and whooping cough (a bacterium in this case) with TB; likewise, vaccinia, the herpes and pox viruses, with Sycosis; finally, glandular fever with cancer.

### THE BOWEL NOSODES[4]
These very valuable remedies, made from cultures of the Salmonellas[b] and related organisms found in the human intestines, seem to be in a somewhat different category, inasmuch as it is the absence of the said organisms that is associated with poor health rather than the reverse. It is as if they serve in the role of 'garbage collectors' and their respective nosodes can perhaps be regarded as the ultimate drainage remedies. But, once again, there are clear relationships between certain of these and the big three.

### SUMMARY SO FAR
It can be postulated, therefore, that TB, the acquired toxins and bowel toxaemia, so-called, would have been parts of the huge complex of disease factors which Hahnemann, for lack of scientific data, was compelled to treat as a single item labelled *Psora*. But having to some extent clarified matters as discussed above, there remains the basic concept of Psora which does not fit into any strict category on its own. We need to consider this in more detail.

# 2

## What is Psora?

The primary aim of homoeopathic treatment is to raise the vitality of the patient, so that he can thereby *'heal himself'*. In modern terms this entails raising the functioning of the integrated adaptive systems known as the *psycho-neuro, endocrine and immune systems* (PNEI),<sup>c</sup> which operate very much as a whole, talking to each other with the same chemical transmitters. If individuals can be successfully treated so that they 'feel better in themselves' i.e., feel that they have more energy, are clearer and calmer mentally and emotionally, it is found that in general their physical ailments start to clear up by themselves. And increased resistance to everyday infections is a common result. Recovery takes place from the inside (from the more vital organs) outwards to less vital organs, and it is often noted that skin eruptions will appear temporarily in the course of this process. This is very clearly seen in the treatment of children with asthma, with a previous history of eczema — the latter will invariably recur as the asthma improves; and the importance of this direction of cure is obvious in that asthma can kill, whereas eczema does not.

The inability to throw out a good rash in, for example, measles, may result in very serious complications, such as convulsions, and the homoeopath could use an antipsoric remedy, probably Cuprum in this instance, to restore the natural course of the illness. By the same token, the external suppression of a skin eruption, or indeed of any other superficial condition, can have the same result, and it was to this aspect that Hahnemann was referring in his original definition of Psora. It can follow, therefore, *from either pre-existing lack of vitality, or from suppression*.

At the psychological level, the same point applies. The suppression or repression of 'hang-ups', whether anxieties, fear, anger, shame, blame or regret, can have dire results. Consider the case of a child who has been abused in some way, and who has been unable, or even not allowed, to talk it out — the result in later life may well be arthritis, colitis, or of course depression, anxiety states, and general emotional and mental dysfunction. What is worse, such dysfunctional states tend to be passed on to others, whether of the same or the next generation, to 'rub off' so to speak, creating more hang-ups and irrational reactions and behaviour patterns, producing the often seen dysfunctional and consequently sick family or group. Nothing is more vitality-depleting than internal suppression of psychological stresses, which leads of course straight into the physical consequences of 'Psora'. In the above would appear to be the explanation of the contagious nature of this first, most basic miasm of all, the *'mother of all diseases'*,[d] and corresponds perfectly with the present-day view that a very high proportion of illness is psycho-somatic in origin.

To quote from Kent's *Lectures on Homoeopathic Philosophy:*[5]

*'The three chronic miasma...are all contagious. In each instance there is something prior to the manifestations we call disease. Psora being the first...it is proper for us to enquire into that state of the human race that would be suitable for the development of Psora...when man began to will the things that were the outcome of his false thinking, he entered a state where...there is evolved from him an aura (which can cause contagion) which is vicious in proportion to his departure from virtue and justice into evils.'*

If one postulates a primitive paradisal state of man, the only two factors that could initiate a fall from such hypothetical perfection would be psychological aberration and/or nutritional imbalance, both being the result of wrong thinking.

From another angle the goal of constitutional homoeopathic treatment is freedom for the individual — freedom from hang-ups and delusions, freedom from the miasmatic/toxic load that we are born with and which, untreated, inexorably increases throughout life, freedom to be creative, freedom to accept and adapt to life with all its attendant and constant changes. It is interesting that the Bach remedy Walnut is used for fear of and inability to adapt to changing life circumstances and, in mythology, walnuts were said to be the food of the gods.

Every hang-up or delusion is thus a denial or suppression in some area of life, a failure of acceptance or openness. Contrast the Buddhist philosophy of the ideal life — simple *awareness* without resistance. Love has been defined as perceptive understanding with consequent absence of criticism or resistance to any situation.[6] So Light (understanding) leads to Love, and where there is Love (non-resistance) there is Life (vitality). It can also be said that where there is vitality there is confidence; where there is confidence there is no feeling of need to resist or suppress, thus there is Love; and where there is Love there is understanding or Light. These three are one; they are simply aspects of the fundamental energy of the Universe, and are the basis of every real religion and every true healing art. In the German language: *heil* means whole or cured; *Heil* means welfare, security; *Heilkunde* is the 'art of healing', and *heilig* means holy. Food for thought!

So the essential nature of Psora is that state of depletion which results, on the one hand, from suppression at any level and, on the other hand, from the depredations of illness — acute or chronic — the mischievous effects of the other miasms, or exertion physically or mentally, injury, poisons (including drugs) and, importantly, also nutritional deficiency. George Vithoulkas describes the Psorinum picture as often the outcome of poverty or deprivation. Essential nutritional elements are typically depleted in illness by being used up in the struggle to survive and, unless replaced, leave a more or less permanent state of lowered resistance to the next assault. This could also be said to apply to a lack of the potency energy, i.e., the correct homoeopathic remedy needed to restore normal functioning. Thus the progression of deteriorating health is a vicious circle — stress of response to infection, circumstances, etc, leading to lowered vitality and less capability of responding adequately to the next stress.

The described characteristics of pure Psora are essentially functional, but the additional presence of other miasms, in practice invariable — no one is naturally free of them — results in the whole plethora of organic diseases with which we are familiar.

## 3

From a practical point of view, since *every* remedy or nosode corresponds with some or other *mis-emotion*, stuck attitude or delusional state,[7,8] it follows that *every* remedy can be regarded as anti-psoric. Many remedies have in fact a broad spectrum of action, and may correspond also with direct effects of the other, *'infective'* miasms. Drosera, for instance, is particularly interesting in that it cures frequently the symptoms of whooping cough; additionally it matches increased susceptibility to tuberculosis and was found (in the days when this still happened) to clear up TB of bone with great efficiency. But it also covers a seriously deranged, paranoid state of mind, actually very similar to that of the late Adolf Hitler.[9] The nosodes seem to have a dual function. They can be prescribed when there are characteristic symptoms, mental and physical, thereby acting in the role of anti-psoric remedies, assisting the patient to throw off the corresponding miasm or toxin. But they can also be used 'isopathically' where there is reason to presume the underlying presence of a miasmatic state, even if the immediate symptoms correspond with a different, related remedy. In fact, while many remedies will clear, for the time being, the *effects* of a miasm, it seems that the nosode is always required at some stage to eradicate the miasm itself. A very common example: Thuja may be needed repeatedly for the effects of smallpox vaccination, but the final clearance of the latter always needs Vaccininum in a high potency. While some homoeopaths dispute the validity of this application of nosodes, in practice, and strongly confirmed by the findings of psionic analysis, it is not only legitimate, but essential.

## Where are the miasms?

How miasms are 'stored' is not really understood. Psora does not come into this part of the discussion, being a dynamic process rather than a toxin or particulate entity. In general, the numerous other miasms and acquired toxins in practice can really be regarded simply as persistent, chronic infections at some level in the organism. In some cases, persistence of actual virus particles occurs as mentioned earlier. In others, particularly the deep inherited miasms, one has to presume a derangement of energy patterns at a non-physical level. In psionic practice, they are found to be associated particularly with DNA and RNA. It seems that, in living systems, every component exists in a number of distinct energetic states, which can be separately examined by using different potencies of the item concerned. Thus certain toxins may be found only for example in $DNA^6$ or $RNA^6$, whereas others may only appear in say $DNA^{12}$ or $DNA^{30}$, etc. Where the toxin is strongly affecting the physical organism, it tends to be picked up at lower levels, whereas a latent or dormant miasm may be found only at the higher potencies.

## Positive or negative response

In examining any diagnostic witness, a positive or negative reaction may be obtained. This is best understood by consideration of the two phases of response by any living organism to any noxious stimulus: at first the phase of reaction; then the phase of exhaustion, and perhaps even death. If one 'flogs a tired horse', the response is at first vigorous flight, then eventually collapse. This sequence is seen, potentially, in every acute illness, though the collapse stage of course occurs only rarely in a healthy subject, unless the virulence of the assault is overwhelming (e.g., meningitis). A positive diagnostic finding corresponds with the phase of reaction — the organism is coping — and the negative with that of exhaustion. It should be obvious to the reader, from what has gone before, that this 'negative phase' is a measure of Psora. Either phase may be found at any level from DNA/RNA through mitochondria (the physical energy generators), all cells throughout the entity, to individual organs or systems. The liver, for instance, in acute hepatitis, will show a positive at Cells³ level. As recovery occurs, this will decrease and disappear, but a residual negative may well be found and remain for some time afterwards, though of course with treatment both phases can be greatly shortened. It is interesting that the phase of exhaustion is so clearly epitomised in the remedy Psorinum — perhaps the most depleted, debilitated, depressed and despairing, chilly and weak remedy in the whole of the Materia Medica — lacking in vitality at every level, and often required after an acute illness.

It is most important in endeavouring to understand the mechanisms of disease to understand that all overreaction — and all perceived symptoms of an inflammatory nature (therefore, 'positive') — can occur only because of an underlying depletion or deficiency of function, at the same or another level, and compensating for the latter. To clarify this, in riding a bicycle one maintains a perfect balance by making tiny adjustments of which one is not even aware. This is the 'state of health'. But if one is partially disabled and has limited capacity for quick reaction, a small disturbance may result in loss of control, followed by a violent over-response and either recovery or disaster. This is the typical experience of the average human in disease. Thus, the fundamental importance of Psora, the underpinning weakness or negative state, is its role in predisposition to every kind of human ill. One should add that chronic degenerative conditions are of course simply persistent and progressive psoric states, albeit brought about by the ravages of stress, suppressions, deficiencies, infections and miasms.

The given symptoms of the remedies of the Homoeopathic Materia Medica, as established by both provings and by cures, may belong in either category — reaction or exhaustion — depending on the extent of the poisoning, or trauma, or infection from which the data was obtained. And, in application, either a remedy or a nosode may be appropriate to treat any state, positive or negative. In the average acute illness, the symptomatic remedy is often facilitated by the additional use of the nosode of the causative organism. Both can be identified or confirmed in most cases by psionic analysis. Chronic diseases require careful progressive elimination of the underlying toxins and miasms, but it cannot be overstressed that the restoration of the depleted, negative psoric states is most fundamental of all. This all-sided approach to healing is the goal of Psionic Medicine.

## Key characteristics of the major miasms

**PSORA:**  Functional disorders. Absence of structural degeneration or disease

Oversensitive. Restless

Mind quick, intelligent

*Anxiety* — disproportionate. Fears

(*Depletion* — resulting from acute disease, activity of other miasms, suppression of physical or emotional states/symptoms)

**SYPHILIS:** Destruction of tissue, deformity, distortion

Ulceration

Neurological disease

Arterial disease. Old age

All congenital abnormalities

Mind slow, stupidity, imbecility

Depression, especially endogenous. Suicidalness

Organic psychoses

<night <sea air > mountains

Accident proneness

'Attract violence'

**TB:**  Overactive. 'Burning up.' 'Consumption.'

Restless, discontented, obstinate

Changeable moods. Changing symptoms

Constantly catching colds, flu, etc

Chesty

Lymphadenopathy

Bone disease. Disorders of calcium metabolism

Allergy (probably). Organic endocrine disease

**SYCOSIS:**   Overgrowth of tissues (→ malignancy)

Chronic disorder of mucous membranes, catarrhs

Urinary disorders. Pelvic disease

Asthma

Rheumatoid arthritis

Early age myocardial infarction

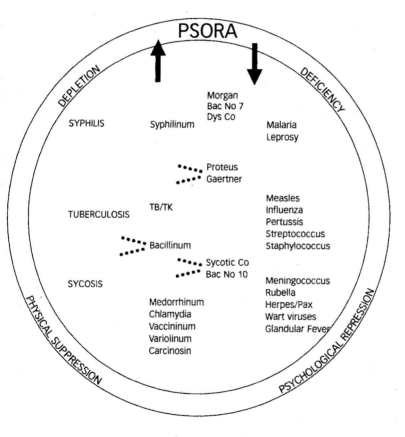

*Figure 9. A schematic representation of miasmatic inter-relationships (suggested, but neither definitive nor complete).*

Mind 'bad': irritability, suspiciousness, jealousy, secretiveness, ddeceitfulness, viciousness. Amoral

< day < damp > sea air

Ailments from birth i.e., first few months of life

Note the following from Figure 9:

- Psora is all-encompassing.
- Psora is both underlying cause and also consequence of the active infective/miasmatic states (hence the arrows going in and out).
- Column 3 contains the bowel nosodes and indicates some relationships.

## References

1. Hahnemann, S.C., *The Chronic Diseases*, 1828
2. Burnett, J.C., *A New Cure of Consumption*, 1906
3. Westlake, A., *A New Dimension in Medicine*, Psionic Medicine Nos 11 & 12, 1976 & 1977
4. Paterson, J., *The Bowel Nosodes*, 1950
5. Kent, J.T., *Lectures on Homoeopathic Philosophy*, No. 19 (reprint 1976)
6. Bailey, A., *Treatise on the Seven Rays*, 1925
7. Sankaran, R., *The Spirit of Homoeopathy* , 1982
8. Kent, J.T., *Repertory of the Homoeopathic Materia Medica — Mind: Anxiety, Fear, Delusions. Sleep: Dreams* (reprint 1986)
9. Shepherd, D., *A Physician's Posy*, C.W. Daniel (Saffron Walden) 1969

## Footnotes

(p. 95) [a]Thus leading to all sorts of quasi-theological arguments as to how everything can be explained as effects of one or the other, or as permutations and combinations of the three.

(p. 97) [b]What would appear to be variants of low or non-virulence are referred to here.

(p. 98) [c]PNEI or PNI –psychoneuroimmunology, see Chapter Three.

(p. 99) [d]The first and last enemy of humanity, 'original sin'.

# The Unitary Theory of Disease

'The third thinker who has helped me evolve a
working philosophy is J.E.R. McDonagh, FRCS.'

**Dr George Laurence**

I t was the conviction that true medicine was concerned with
causes rather than clinical symptoms that prompted George
Laurence to stretch his mind beyond the limits of ordinary
acceptance. He began to investigate unconventional techniques,
not from a purely theoretical standpoint, but as a method of rein-
forcing his well-established orthodox knowledge. But with a characteristic blend of caution and intuition he did not pin his faith to
any one system, believing that all these methods were comple-
mentary facets of an underlying truth. Hence, if we are to follow
his quest we must also consider a variety of aspects of causal
medicine, which may at first appear to be unconnected, but
which will ultimately be seen to be integrated within the overall
pattern.

## The 'Great Triumvirate'[1]

Laurence acknowledged the influence of three great thinkers in
his search for the truth. The first of these was Samuel Hahnemann,
whose concept of illness as a result of disturbance of the Vital
Force corresponded with Laurence's intuitive intimations of reality.

The second was Rudolph Steiner, whose concept of the etheric
world confirmed the possibility of influences and causes of a

superior order, and whose notion of Formative Forces provided a further reinforcement for Laurence's own developing theories.

It was while he was at this stage of his work that he came in contact with his third source of inspiration, in the person of J.E.R. McDonagh, FRCS, with whom he had a number of discussions. McDonagh had been pursuing the idea that all disease arose from a derangement of the vital energies in the body.

## McDonagh's Unitary Theory

McDonagh believed the vital energies to be responsible for the formation of proteins, which are the essential building blocks of all living matter, so that any disturbance of the vital harmony caused a corresponding aberration in the protein production. Hence he maintained that there was only one basic disease, which arose from some imbalance in the protein structure. The clinical symptoms, whatever their nature and classification, by implication would be evidence of malfunction of some part of the intricate mechanisms of the body, arising entirely from an aberration of the protein. So although these symptoms can be studied in great detail, and the conditions partially ameliorated by palliative techniques of various kinds, no real cure would be possible unless the underlying protein imbalance could be redressed.

The extent of this aberration would determine the seriousness of the disorder. Indeed, McDonagh suggested that malignant disease was the result of an extreme degree of protein imbalance, making it a constitutional malady and not just a local disturbance.

This is a very simplified statement of what is known as the *Unitary Theory of Disease*, a very significant concept which has never been universally accepted.[2] We shall discuss it in more detail shortly, but it is evident that *it provides a good model for the way in which the etheric and physical levels may be linked*.

If the primary cause of illness is a disharmony of the vital energies, one can understand that this can be manifest in physical terms as an imbalance of the protein structure, resulting in the clinical symptoms of disease. Laurence intuitively recognised the practical possibilities of this concept and was able by patient experimentation to utilise it in developing the integrated technique of diagnosis and treatment, which has become the basis of Psionic Medicine.

## Maya and the Breath of Brahma

McDonagh's ideas were ahead of their time, unacceptable to orthodox materialism which found his detailed formulations difficult, and even fanciful. Yet his basic concept is entirely compatible with modern scientific thought which, as we have seen, regards matter as a local condensation of an all-pervading energy pattern (see Chapter Two, by Professor Ervin Laszlo, on the Psi-Field Hypothesis).

It is clear that we live in a world of illusion in which the very building blocks of our material universe, the molecules, atoms and subatomic particles, have an indeterminate physical existence. They are moving, coming in and out of existence, and we have no control whatsoever over them. This world of illusion, in Hindu philosophy, is termed *Maya*.

We live in Maya, because that is generally all that we can deal with. We are aware of atoms and molecules, and the transience of some of these incredible subatomic particles, yet in day to day existence they seem an academic abstraction. We do not think of what is happening to individual atoms as we write, eat, play golf or stroke a cat. Similarly, in our perception of the way our body works, or fails to work, we do not tend to think of what is happening at the subatomic or atomic levels.

In terms of ordinary sense-based intelligence (in the world of Maya) these more refined implications are unnecessary. It is possible to cope adequately with material problems by the application of conventional knowledge. But it is obvious that sense-based awareness and conventional knowledge (in terms of the conventionally understood five senses) is of a strictly limited character, and particularly in its medical aspects falls far short of true understanding. If we are to surmount this barrier it is necessary to relate our thinking to the concepts of the real world, and specifically to the pattern of the etheric realm in which the true causes and relationships exist.

The concept which McDonagh was coming to was very much of a dynamic state of affairs involving repeated cycles of growth and repair. Hence he did not consider the physical world to be a permanent crystallisation of the etheric fabric, but to be continuously created by rhythmic condensations of the etheric force field in successively more complex form.

This concept is entirely consistent with esoteric cosmology, which regards the universe as a living entity animated by a continual flow and return of energy, called in Hindu philosophy the *Breath of Brahma*. And as we have seen before, there are great similarities with the Psi-Field Hypothesis.

## Successive cycles of complexity

This was the idea that McDonagh endeavoured to develop in support of his Unitary Theory of Disease. He formulated the concept in considerable detail, notably in a series of writings on the nature of disease but, because this involved new directions of thought in advance of accepted ideas, his theories met with little recognition, and even provoked hostility. Moreover, this very detail tended to obscure the essential simplicity of his vision: namely that it was possible for these ordered processes to become deranged and that it was these aberrations from the norm which produced the symptoms of disease.

It was this aspect of the idea which Laurence intuitively recognised as providing the integrating factor in his study of the imbalance of vital energy and which he was then able to apply to provide a practical system of therapy.

So let us now look at the basis of McDonagh's theory. It helps to consider several cycles of increasing complexity.

Briefly, McDonagh postulated a 'primordial activity' (which we can consider to be the psi-field), from which the matter-energies of the physical world are formed by a series of pulsations in an evolutionary spiral. The first stage creates the subatomic particles of almost negligible half-life, but which are continually replenished.

The second cycle is concerned with the integration of these particles into atoms, forming three distinct (unequal) groups performing specific functions, which he calls radiation, attraction and storage. One could think of this as being akin to the metallic elements playing an active role, which would be compatible with McDonagh's concept of a radiative function, the basic elements exercising an attractive function, and the inert gases exhibiting a storage function.

The third cycle involves the formation of the simple molecules and their arrangement in the crystalline structures which constitute the basis of inorganic matter. Here again the compounds, according to their nature, exercise one of the three specific functions which determine their quality in the overall chemical structure.

There then follows a fourth cycle concerned with the more elaborate molecular structures of so-called organic compounds. These include the colloids, such as albumen, and the amino acids, which are the building blocks of protein, the essential constituent of living matter. There appears at this stage to be an infusion of vital energy — possibly the *Vis Medicatrix Naturae* — which permits the molecules to exercise all three primary functions in an appropriate degree, instead of only one as with the inorganic compounds.

From this develops a fifth cycle in which the proteins are elaborated into the various interdependent structures of the vegetable world, followed by the sixth cycle concerned with the requirements of the animal kingdom in which the proteins are diversified into the tissues and organs of the body.

According to McDonagh, life is sustained by the continuous pulsation of vital energy in the essential proteins, each of which must provide an appropriate and harmonious exercise of the functions of radiation, attraction and storage. It is thus plausible that if this essential rhythm is disturbed by some extraneous influence

— such as miasms and toxins — this will produce a condition of disease, accompanied by clinical symptoms of varying severity.

## Commentary by George Laurence on McDonagh's Unitary Concept of Disease in Relation to Radiesthetic Diagnosis

*(An original paper by Dr George Laurence, delivered to the Medical Society for Medical Radiesthesia)*

'The essence of McDonagh's theory is that there is only one disease, and that it arises from the protein in the blood being so affected that it can no longer properly fulfil its original function of attracting food, storing it in itself, and then radiating it to the tissues and organs in a balanced way.

'All so-called diseases are merely manifestations of imbalance or aberration of the protein, and no disease can be cured unless that balance is restored. McDonagh points out that you may palliate or alleviate manifestations of disease, you can suppress and drive them from one place to another (e.g., the alternation of skin disease and asthma as the result of treatment directed solely to one or the other manifestation), and you can keep them hidden for long periods, but you cannot cure them unless you can find the basic cause or common denominator. However perfect a chemotherapeutic preparation may be, it can never be relied upon to remove all the lesions and effect the disappearance of all such manifestations, as its sole action is to repair the local secondary damage suffered by the protein; and as it has no effect whatsoever upon the primary cause or causes of the damage, that repair may be of a very temporary nature. This is a point of importance which orthodox medicine seems to be generally sublimely oblivious — or indifferent!

'The real question before us is: *why is there a primary protein imbalance?*

'Infection by micro-organisms may come to mind and steps be taken to destroy them biochemically; but in killing them, have you found the reason why the individual became in the first place so vulnerable to attack? Why is health so undermined as to permit the invasion? Or again, as many of us are beginning to wonder, what is amiss with our mental and spiritual outlook, or with our food and environment, that the resistance of our tissues is so low?

'To get nearer the answer to our question it seems necessary to consider the nature of health; and to arrive at this we must realise that an important part of its origin lies in the soil. Micro-organisms, by their action on other micro-organisms and the mineral and plant life, liberate vital energies which constitute the principal ingredient of the nourishment extracted by plants from the soil. Hence a deficiency of life in the soil means inferiority of food for animals, and so for men, whether taken in animal or vegetable form.

'To quote McDonagh, "The soil beneath our feet is not simply a dead, inert mass, but is composed of countless millions of living organisms, each with its own tiny life cycle and particular work to perform. Healthy vital bodies require vital foods grown upon living soil. Yet what do we find? Sick bodies and minds and uncontrolled emotions, fed upon devitalised foods which have been raised upon sick, tired and worn-out soil."

'Thus an important factor of health is the state of the soil and there is a link here with protein aberrations in the body. It is encouraging to note, therefore, that the question of soil is at last getting some consideration particularly in regard to the deficiencies that we have to contend with in treatment of both acute and chronic disease.

'Climate and proper food are the fundamental requirements for the soil and its micro-organisms, and when conditions exist such as an unsuitable climate, exhaustion of the soil or ill-treatment by chemical fertilisers or insecticides and weedkillers, the micro-organisms are unable to do their work properly and thus our food suffers. We have no control over climate and, as individuals, very little over the quality of the food that is offered to us, but we can be more careful in our choice of food. If the public demand for wholemeal flour, brown sugar and cereals, fruit and vegetables grown on compost-cultivated soil, clean milk, unadulterated and genuine food, became sufficiently loud and powerful (and was listened to and acted upon), there would be an enormous decrease in chronic disease and an improvement in the health of the nation.

'In addition to the intestinal toxaemia caused by contaminated and unsuitable food, there are, of course, a large number of other causes of chronic disease — occupational, psychological and environmental — to which must be added the debilitating effects of the miasms. All of these influences create disturbance of the balance of protein so that in this sense there is, as McDonagh affirms, only one disease.'

'McDonagh maintains that under the influence of 'climate', which I understand to mean cosmic energy, all protein alternately expands and contracts, and if the extent and rhythm of this pulsation is upset — rendered aberrant, to use his own term — you have a state of imbalance and the condition necessary to produce disease.

'He divides protein into three portions corresponding to and exercising the three main developmental divisions of the body. These he calls the *Epiblast*, the *Mesoblast* and the *Hypoblast*, which should operate in harmony.

'Very briefly, McDonagh derives from the *mesoblast*:

Musculoskeletal system
Cardiovascular system
Genitourinary system
Adrenal cortex

from the *hypoblast*:

Blood
Respiratory system
Thyroid
Portal system

from the *epiblast*:

Adrenal medulla
Anterior pituitary
Posterior pituitary
Sympathetic nervous system
Parasympathetic nervous system

'In any disease, the actual symptoms may differ according to which portions of the protein are most thrown out of balance, but as you cannot confine a toxin to one portion of the body, you generally have to deal with the whole picture in the first place.

## Pendulum diagnosis

'From a sample of the patient, such as a spot of blood, saliva or hair, a considerable amount of information about the state of protein can be obtained by the use of the pendulum in experienced hands — quite unbelievable, of course, to the uninitiated and orthodox fraternity; this I can well understand, for when I first heard of radiesthesia, I was similarly sceptical. But the technique is now scientifically established, and I find it sad that so many people are suffering unnecessarily for want of informed treatment beyond the scope of the more or less casual administration of synthetic chemicals, so many of which are poisonous because they cause further imbalance of the protein; and this despite the fact that they can produce only temporary alleviation or suppression of symptoms.

'By the use of the pendulum it is possible to find out, with the aid of samples and witnesses, whether a toxin is present, what it is and its extent, and what particular part of the body is mostly being affected. As a poison cannot be confined to one place (think of a snake bite, or even a sting), it is neither sensible nor even intelligent to treat any specific effect before removing the cause. Once you have dealt with the primary cause, you can treat such symptoms as are still left with the ordinary homoeopathic remedies and so redress any secondary aberration of the protein in the individual organs.

'The principle of first finding the basic cause of any malady applies with special force to chronic disease. I could give many examples of this, but an outstanding one is afforded by many cases of alternating asthma and eczema, which I have seen during some sixty years of practice. Both chest specialists and dermatologists can give temporary relief to one or other manifestation, often causing an exacerbation of the untreated symptom, but neither knowing what is really the matter with the patient nor ascertaining the basic cause.

'It seems to me quite wrong to accept a name or a label as a true diagnosis. Surely that term should include the cause; otherwise it can only claim to be a provisional diagnosis. Another example is migraine, the treatment of which seems to be much on the same lines as when I was a student, whereas the underlying cause can be different in different people. Until that cause is removed, you can again only expect temporary relief by drugs — with the very definite risk of serious side effects.

'So many of these chronic diseases are due to inherited miasms or acquired toxins which remain in the body, and these can only be detected by supersensory methods. The outlook for the effective handling of such cases appears to be very grim, unless the value of psionic techniques for diagnosis and treatment becomes more widely recognised.

'It is little short of amazing how, with a little practice, the pendulum will pick out the appropriate remedy, and moreover tell you quite definitely which potency is likely to be the most effective. This is of special value as, in orthodox homoeopathic teaching, the question of potencies is always a stumbling block and depends very much on the personal preference or experience of the practitioner. Furthermore, the pendulum can give you a very good idea of the exact dosage and the length of time for which the remedy should be prescribed.

'To recapitulate, the basic structure of the body consists of protein, for which fats and carbohydrates act mostly as fuel. Any condition that disturbs the harmonious balance of the protein causes ill health, of which the manifestations and symptoms depend upon what region or regions of the protein are suffering the imbalance.

'In my own practice the great proportion of cases, before I see them, have been subjected to the most exhaustive — and often exhausting — investigations: clinical, laboratory, Barium meals,

X-rays, etc., with negative results, and patients have come to see me as a last hope. It is quite wonderful how frequently psionic techniques will provide not only a true diagnosis, but also an effective treatment, especially in the case of the so-called incurable diseases, of which the basic cause has so seldom been found.

'I should like to say a word at this juncture about potencies. By potentising a substance you are transforming it into energy, which acts at a much higher level of intensity than can be effected by crude drugs. In a sense you are making the substance radioactive,[3] for it is through this 'activity' or radiative effect that the remedy acts, meanwhile retaining the influence or character of the original drug substance. Nothing can be compared to this radiative effect of potentised remedies for the elimination of miasms and toxins, or indeed for correcting imbalances in the protein.

'I owe a debt of gratitude to McDonagh for the light he has thrown on the problem of medicine and very much regret that so few orthodox doctors will even try to understand what he means by his Unitary Theory, much less apply it to the elucidation of the problem of disease and use it for the alleviation of human suffering.'

Psionic practitioners today are conscious of the role of protein aberration in the causation of illness. As indicated in the last chapter by Dr Farley Spink, the present Dean of the Institute of Psionic Medicine, one's investigations can range far and wide. One may look at tissues, cells, DNA, RNA, virtually any cellular component, including the mitochondrion, and one may have to look at each at different energy levels. Suffice it to say that McDonagh's insights opened up new vistas of investigation.

---

[1] In ancient Rome, a *triumvir* was one of three men united in office. The first *Great Triumvirate* in 60BC was formed between Pompey, Julius Caesar and Crassus.
[2] This chapter has been left almost unchanged, because of its historical importance as one of the main influences upon Laurence. Most current Psionic Practitioners would accept some aspects of the theory rather than its totality.
[3] Laurence is not saying that the potentisation of a remedy makes it radioactive in the scientifically accepted sense. He is using this in a metaphorical sense.

# Intuition, Extra-Sensory Perception and Psi Phenomena

*'If the doors of perception were cleansed everything would appear, as it is, infinite.'*

**William Blake (1757–1827)**

Several references have been made in the preceding chapters to the existence of paranormal senses which are responsible for the faculty usually called intuition: and since the psionic diagnosis and treatment of the underlying causes of disease involve the scientific use of these faculties it is desirable to discuss the nature and possibilities of these paranormal senses in some detail.

We have already established that the physical world of everyday experience is only an interpretation, by a strictly limited range of senses, of an incredibly complicated universe. The building bricks of that universe are not, as we have seen, as substantial as we once believed them to be. And indeed, with the psi-field hypothesis we begin to understand that there is reality in the concept of the interconnected universe, which has always been recognised by the shaman, the mystic and the enlightened of many cultures throughout history.

Man is, however, provided with a range of additional senses, which respond to impressions of a different quality, which are not detected by the conventional senses. These are the paranormal senses, meaning that they exist side by side with the normal physical senses. There are people in whom these latent faculties are unusually developed, which tends to create the belief that they are in some way abnormal. But this is incorrect, for these additional senses are part of man's normal equipment. It just happens that because they are unused they have become dormant.

With our preoccupation with material phenomena we take the physical senses completely for granted, and fail to realise that we have had to be educated to interpret their responses. A similar education and cultivation is necessary to exercise the paranormal senses, but this we do not normally find necessary because we can cope quite adequately with the world of facts by the processes of logical reasoning.

Nevertheless, we have cursory awareness of these paranormal responses, which manifest themselves in what is customarily called 'sensitivity'. We instinctively like or dislike people or places. We recognise that certain situations are right, without being able to say why. Let us look at some of these strange 'feelings' and see how they can lead to a deeper awareness of our paranormal senses.

## Gut feelings, rules of thumb and sixth sense

Virtually everyone will have experienced a so-called 'gut feeling' at some time or another. For some reason, which they are unable to rationalise, they will have had an absolute conviction that something is right or wrong, or that they should take a particular course of action. And in the majority of occasions that they experience this gut feeling, they will subsequently find that the feeling was correct.

Many people also employ an heuristic approach in their decision-making. Heuristics[1] are essentially 'rules of thumb'. Carpenters, mechanics, doctors, businessmen — indeed, most people in busy occupations — will use rules of thumb to sort out problems. Psychologists have shown that although three broad mental levels may be brought to the task — skill-base, rule-base and knowledge-base — they will still often arrive at a decision using a rule of thumb.

It is quite analogous to doing mental arithmetic. Faced with a complicated piece of multiplication and division, most people will perform an estimate first to lead them to the solution. But sometimes the decision reached can be extremely accurate. It is as if some other sophistication is brought into the heuristic approach from some other, unknown, source.

And then there is the *sixth sense* phenomenon. This is actually very common in medicine. One often hears, usually anecdotally, about someone making a very sharp diagnosis on a patient, despite having scant or insufficient data. It sometimes happens even when the patient has very little to complain about, yet the doctor just knows that there is something significantly wrong. It is usually jokingly written off as being the doctor's 'sixth sense', but inwardly the individual is congratulating him or herself upon their cleverness or the astuteness of their diagnostic acumen. In a profession which prides itself on being 'clever', because every case has to have a diagnosis or solution, an heuristic approach is considered acceptable, especially if it is backed up by the explanation that 'experience teaches you to sense these things'.

Well, this may be the case, but equally well it could be an instance whereby the doctor is allowing a higher sense to come into play. This, one suspects, goes beyond heuristics, or at least further than heuristics are usually deemed to go. Or, then again, perhaps heuristics is a way of permitting that higher sense to come into play. Perhaps because we are so firmly in the age of rationalism, of so-called *'evidence-based science and medicine'*, we deny those higher senses?

If so, we are possibly denying an important part of our being.

## Extra-sensory perception and psychokinesis

There have been reports of paranormal phenomena in virtually every culture since the beginnings of recorded history. Indeed, referring back to Sir James Frazer's[2] concept that society advances through the phases of magic, religion and science, such phenomena have in turn been rationalised as magic, miracles or paranormal events. Of course, in the phase of science there is a tendency to write such phenomena off as superstition, coincidence or fraud, yet the very fact that people are aware of them, that they are considered outwith normal and everyday events means that there is a legitimate (and necessary) reason to study them.

The first systematic study of these phenomena began in 1882, when the Society for Psychical Research was founded in London by the philosopher, Henry Sedgwick. His co-founders were the physicists Sir Oliver Lodge,[3] Sir William Barrett and Sir William Crookes, and the philosophers Frederick W.H. Myers and Edmund Gurney. In 1885, following a meeting between Sedgwick and the psychologist William James, a twin organisation came into being with the founding of the American Society for Psychical Research. The early focus of research for both societies was in the growing field of spiritualism and mediumship.

The first effective scientific research into psychic phenomena began in the 1920s, under the direction of Professor Joseph B. Rhine (1895–1980) in the psychology department at Duke University, North Carolina. Rhine had received his doctorate in plant physiology in 1925 from the University of Chicago, but in 1926 he and his wife, Louisa E. Rhine,[4] joined William McDougall at Harvard. When McDougall moved to Duke University in 1927 they followed him and, at his instigation in 1930, began a series of experiments on psychic phenomena. This was to be the beginning of a new branch of psychology.

Rhine took a quite different approach from the early psychic researchers by studying 'everyday' people rather than professed psychics. His hypothesis was that if psychic abilities exist, then they should be apparent within the general population. Accordingly, his first subjects were recruited from the student body at Duke.

Initially, Rhine wanted to study telepathic ability using playing cards. It became clear to him, however, that 52 separate 'symbols' were possibly too many to deal with, but that some subjects might subconsciously over-select favourite cards or reject particular numbers which they were superstitious about. A colleague, Karl Zenner, came up with the solution by producing a deck of twenty-five cards, consisting of five cards each of five different symbols. These were: a square, a circle, a star, a set of wavy lines, and a plus sign.

In the classic Rhine experiments the subject tries to perceive the order of the five symbols when they are randomly shuffled. Since the chance of predicting a symbol is one in five, it is a relatively easy matter to calculate the probability of achieving particular scores. Sometimes the experiments were conducted facing the subject over a table, sometimes in a different room and sometimes in different buildings.

Rhine found some subjects were particularly adept with the Zenner cards, consistently producing results which were statistically significant. In 1934 he published his research in a monograph entitled *Extra-Sensory Perception*. His choice of the term had been carefully made, since he postulated that the perception was outwith the usual five senses.

An interesting phenomenon which Rhine commented upon was 'missing ESP'. This can be thought of as a sort of 'reverse ESP', whereby some subjects would consistently do worse than chance. It was postulated that these individuals may block out any perception, possibly through unconscious negativity.

Also in 1934, Rhine devised a series of dice tests to study the phenomenon of *psychokinesis* (PK), the apparent influence of mind over matter, or the ability to 'will' objects to move. Here, again, Rhine's early results with a gambler who claimed to be able to influence falling dice seemed to be significantly greater than chance. But Rhine was justifiably cautious about publishing his results, and it was not until 1943 that his controversial findings were released to the scientific community.

Rhine believed that ESP and PK were two phenomena, which were not connected to any physical component of the brain. He felt that neither could be explained by the known laws of physics, but that nonetheless they were real, observable and demonstrable phenomena.

## Psi and parapsychology

In 1946 Dr Robert Thouless and his colleague, Dr W.P. Weisner suggested that *Psi* (the twenty-third letter of the Greek alphabet — Ψ) should be used as a designation for ESP and PK, because both phenomena seem to be closely related.

J.B. Rhine is credited with naming the new discipline for the study of psi phenomena *'parapsychology'*, from the Greek *'para'*, meaning beyond.[5]

The Rhines were the most famous of the parapsychologists up until the 1960s and, since they were responsible for training many researchers, their influence has been long-lasting. In addition to helping her husband's work, Louisa Rhine performed major research on spontaneous ESP and spontaneous PK.

In 1965 Rhine retired from Duke University and moved his research lab off campus. In a modified form as the Rhine Research Center's Institute for Parapsychology it is still making major contributions to the field.

During the 1960s mainstream psychology was focussing attention upon the nature of consciousness. Understandably, parapsychologists then started looking at the nature of psychological processes involved in psi. This saw the development of 'process-oriented' psi research, or studies on the manner in which psi can be affected by time, distance, state of consciousness (and therefore altered states of consciousness), and by personal factors such as mood, personality and attitude to psi. Testing became for *'free-response'* ESP, rather than previous testing *by 'forced choice'*, as in the classic Zenner-card predictions.

A major research program on dream ESP was established by Montague Ullman and Stanley Krippner at the Maimonides Hospital in Brooklyn, New York, which ran through the 1960s and 1970s. When the program ended in 1979, Charles Honorton,[6] a member of the Maimonides team, opened a new laboratory in

Princeton, New Jersey. There, he continued the free-response work using sensory deprivation conditions called 'ganzfeld' stimulation.[7]

Another major research program began in 1972 at the Stanford Research Institute in California under the direction of physicists Harold Puthoff, Russell Targ and Edwin May. They concentrated on *'remote viewing'* research and became well-known for their high-tech studies of brain function during psi, using such tools as magnetoencephalographs.

There are currently more than 100 universities and research institutes worldwide involved in parapsychological research. The first Chair of Parapsychology was established after World War II at Utrecht University in the Netherlands, the first professor being W.H.C. Tenhaeff. In 1985, the Koestler Chair of Parapsychology was established at the University of Edinburgh, the first holder being Professor Robert L. Morris.

The range of subjects under research nowadays is quite large, but broadly speaking may be looked at under three themes:

- *ESP* — Extra-sensory perception, including telepathy, remote viewing, clairvoyance, clairaudience, clairsentience, (respectively, seeing, hearing and feeling paranormal phenomena), radiesthesia and dowsing

- *PK* — Psychokinesis, literally the influence of mind over matter. Two classes are generally considered: *micro-PK*, which results in weak or very slight effects which are not visible to the naked eye and which may require statistical evaluation, e.g., influencing dice; *macro-PK*, which results in observable phenomena, such as metal bending and levitation

- *Survival issues* — to do with the survival of spirit beyond death or outside the body. Thus, reincarnation, near-death experiences (NDE),[8] out-of-body experiences (OBE), channelling and karma

There are many theories about the mechanism of psi, which is understandable because people come to study parapsychology from many different disciplines. Thus there are psychological theories, physical theories, sociological and psychophysical theories. Inevitably, there is much debate.

## The collective unconscious

The Swiss psychiatrist, Carl C. Jung (1875–1961), had been greatly influenced by Sigmund Freud between the years 1907 to 1913. However, Jung rejected Freud's view that the unconscious was purely personal, and formed of repressed childhood traumas. Instead, Jung believed that, beneath consciousness, there was a personal unconscious, but that beneath that there was a collective unconscious.

The collective unconscious, in Jung's view, was inborn, neither made up of personal experience, nor inherited from one's forebears. It was literally universal.

One can immediately see an analogy in Jung's collective unconscious with the *Akashic Records* referred to in Theosophy. These, according to theosophical teachings, are the master records of everything that has ever occurred since the beginning of the universe. The term comes from the Sanskrit '*Akasha*' which means the 'ether', or the all-pervasive space. Theosophists believe that a vibrational record exists on the astral plane of every sound, light, thought, action and emotion.

Edgar Cayce (1877–1945), the famous American psychic and healer, became famous for his trance-readings. During these trances, which he began doing in 1901 after having been taught how to induce a self-hypnotic trance by hypnotist Al Layne, Cayce consulted the Akashic Records which he sometimes also called the '*Universal Memory of Nature*' or the '*Book of Life*'. Apparently he used a visual technique whereby he would picture a library containing a huge number of books, each of which contained the life story of a person. In order to help someone, all he had to do was find the appropriate book, open it and read the necessary remedy.

At about the same time Rudolph Steiner (1861–1925) was also accessing the Akashic Records, which he termed the *Akashic Chronicle*.

Both these men claimed that the records were open to all who cared to view them, that they were universal, and that it was merely a matter of finding a way of accessing them.

### The psi-field

The psi-field, a universal information field, fulfils all of the concepts that we have discussed. One can see how it accommodates the Akashic Records, the collective unconscious, the morphic or morphogenetic field and the other facets we discussed in our model in Chapter Four. One can see how it allows for the phenomenon of spontaneous culture linkage (see Chapter One), as well as accounting for the phenomena of ESP, transpersonal connections and possibly many survival effects.

Whether reincarnation[9] actually occurs or not, the psi-field hypothesis offers an explanation for past-life recall. The personal psi-field of one individual growing in their mother's womb may, for want of another word, 'vibrate' in an identical, or near identical, way with the recorded personal psi-field of someone who has died. The psi-field of the living and developing individual may then have the ability to unlock the record of experiences, the memories of that other person. They would become incorporated within their mind, their field as 'their own' memories and experiences, albeit from a former existence or incarnation.

### Dowsing

Dowsing is a means of accessing the psi-field. Put very simply, it is an altered state of consciousness in which part of the mind is almost allowed to go to sleep so that the unconscious mind can be contacted. The unconscious thereby allows an ideomotor response to indicate answers to questions which are formulated by the alert half of the mind. We shall consider this more completely in the next chapter.

J.H. Reyner, the principal author of the first edition of this book, had this to say:

'*It remains to consider how the paranormal senses can communicate with the relationships existing in the real world. Here we can be assisted by Swedenborg's[10] concept of "time-body".[11] This again I have discussed in detail in one of my former books,* The Diary of a Modern Alchemist, *but we can review the idea briefly in terms of what has already been postulated. We have seen that the appearances of the physical world are a translation of the successive manifestations in time of a superior and relatively eternal fabric in the real world. This means that the progress of events in the phenomenal world leaves a permanent (though not unalterable) trace in the real world, which is called the "time-body". All the events, and physical conditions, of life thus have their counterpart in the etheric world as a pattern which continues to exist when the finger of time has moved on, so that the transitory situations of life are merely a translation by the physical senses of a much greater and permanent entity in the real world.*

'*This is a concept of enormously expanded potentialities. It not only confirms the idea previously mentioned that the physical body is only a small part of the real structure but, even more significantly, it is applicable to the whole of the phenomenal world, so that every object in the familiar world has its own time-body which extends in the realm of eternity far beyond its transitory appearance. Moreover, this time-body will include everything that has happened to it during its lifetime, which may be much longer than the human life span.*

'*This is sometimes interpreted by saying that every object in nature contains its own intrinsic (intangible) vibrations. It is simpler, however, to conceive it in terms of the time-body, which contains the whole history of the object,* and its associations. *This is an important corollary, for the etheric world,[12] in which the time-body resides, is essentially a pattern of relationships, within which there are many connections, which are not apparent to conventional observation. The paranormal senses, which are of a superior order, can respond to impressions emanating from any part of the time-body, and so assess the real causes and situations behind the physical manifestations.*

'It is thus possible to understand how information as to the real condition of a patient can be obtained from a blood spot or similar sample. The physical constitution of the sample is unimportant, its significance being that it establishes a link between the mind of the practitioner and the time-body of the patient; and hence its influence is not confined to the moment in time when it was originally supplied, but can provide information about subsequent conditions.

'This link between the mind of the dowser and the situation under examination is an essential requirement of the technique (which cannot be mechanised). One has to hold in mind the patient, or situation, under consideration and then formulate a specific question, discarding utterly any preconceived notions, when a clear and unequivocal answer is obtained, if the question has been correctly framed.'

'One of the aspects which is, at first, difficult to understand is the ability to communicate with a person, or a situation, at a distance, or in some other part of passing time. To appreciate this we must remember that the time-body contains a permanent record of the unmanifest pattern, including all its subtle interconnections with other time-bodies; and the quiet mind of the experienced dowser can communicate with any part of this real fabric, provided that he has some sample to serve as a focus for his thoughts.'

## Map dowsing

'As a practical example of the extraordinary possibilities which exist we may refer to the practice of map dowsing, which is quite inexplicable in conventional terms. An experienced dowser can locate water or other deposits by using his pendulum on a map of the locality, subsequently confirming the indications by inspection of the actual site. This is particularly useful in archaeological research, where it is possible to examine the map of an area suspected of containing the buried remains of Roman or other civilisations. If this proves positive, a local search is made, often with surprisingly accurate results.

'Now while one can understand that the time-body of the original Roman villa or other structure continues to exist in the etheric world, including its subsequent history through the intervening centuries, its connection with a modern map seems more obscure. The map, of course, is a reproduction, maybe many times removed, of an actual survey of the site, and thereby contains a tenuous contact with the etheric pattern; but its main significance is that it serves as a focus for the mind of the dowser, whereby his paranormal senses can establish communication with the time-body of the actual locality.

'This is an example of the subtle interconnections which exist in the etheric world. The time-body of an object or location is not confined to the physical entity but includes everything with which it has been connected throughout its existence. We often refer to a house as having a pleasant (or evil) "atmosphere". This intuitive feeling is an unconscious exercise of the paranormal sense, which is aware of the emotional influences of its former inhabitants. The stones of a cathedral are impregnated with the influences not only of the original masons, but also of the thousands of worshippers who have used it subsequently. Similarly, the quality of any work of art or music is determined not merely by its creator, but by all its subsequent history and experiences.

'Psionic Medicine is concerned with more immediate influences extending normally over a few generations only. Its significance lies in the fact that by the use of the normally dormant paranormal senses it is possible, practically and scientifically, to communicate with the time-body of a patient, and provide effective treatment, if necessary, of any aberrations disclosed.'

[1]Heuristic, from the Greek *Heurisko*, meaning 'find'.
[2]Sir James Frazer's *The Golden Bough*, referred to in Chapter One.

[3]Sir Oliver Lodge, Professor of Physics at Liverpool University, an early influence on Dr George Laurence.

[4]Louisa E. Rhine (1891–1983), wife of J.B. Rhine, but a leading parapsychologist in her own right. She was the foremost student of spontaneous psi in her era.

[5]J.B. Rhine actually adopted the term 'parapsychology' from the German term 'parapsychologie', which had been introduced in the late nineteenth century by philosopher-psychologist, Max Dessoir.

[6]Sadly, Charles Honorton died tragically in 1992 at the early age of 46, while undertaking a PhD at the University of Edinburgh.

[7]Ganzfeld, from the German for 'whole field', is a procedure designed to damp down all external sensory stimulation so that the subject can focus attention on thoughts and impressions. The subject lies quietly while 'white noise' is played through earphones and the eyes are covered with shades.

[8]David Lorimer, a NDE researcher describes two kinds of near-death recall. The first is *panoramic memory*, whereby the individual experiences a display of images and memories but without any emotional experience. The second is the *life-review*, wherein life flashes past, but emotions are felt and some moral judgement is made.

[9]Reincarnation has been an accepted tenet of many religions throughout history. Roughly 60 per cent of people globally believe in some form of reincarnation. Hinduism and Buddhism both accept it, as do many tribal societies. It is often linked to the concept of karma.

[10]Emmanuel Swedenborg (1689–1772), Swedish scientist, engineer, statesman, and philosopher. He claimed to experience contacts with other realms of being, usually in a state of consciousness. From these he constructed a complete cosmogony of the other realms in relation to that of the physical.

[11]Swedenborg's 'time-body' seems to be the same as the personal psi-field.

[12]For the 'etheric world' consider the psi-field.

# PART TWO

# THE HISTORY
## AND PRACTICE OF
### PSIONIC MEDICINE

# The History of Dowsing and Radiesthesia

'History is philosophy from examples.'

**Dionysius of Halicarnassus (fl.30–7 BC)**

L et us begin by looking at what we mean by these terms. Dowsing is the name for the practice of finding things by relying upon the movement of some inanimate object which is held in the hands of the operator. As such it is the collective name for a number of diverse practices ranging from simple water-divining, which is really only water-detecting, to the practice of map reading, the location of missing persons, and diagnosis and treatment of illness. Many groups of people may claim to dowse, though they may have completely different concepts both of what dowsing is and how it works.

*Radiesthesia* is the name for the study of the dowsing phenomenon. Whereas *dowsing* basically accepts and does not imply a questioning of the nature of the phenomenon, radiesthesia attempts to explain and advance the subject as a scientific discipline. The word radiesthesia was first coined by the French Abbé Alexis Bouley from the Latin *radiare*, meaning ray or emission of rays, and the Greek *aisthanesthai*, meaning to perceive.

As such the original implication was that in some way the individual perceives something which emanates like a radiation from the object under study.

Dowsing is an art, which stretches back at least to the days of the ancient Egyptians. Tomb paintings clearly illustrate priests using forked sticks to dowse. Similarly, artefacts from ancient China prove that the divining rod was known and used in the imperial courts. Going even further back, Neolithic cave paintings discovered in NW Africa are suggestive of the use of dowsing as long ago as 7–8,000 years ago.

Virtually all civilisations have used skilled dowsers to discover water, precious ores and minerals. Some adepts even extended the range of dowsing activities to aid the law in the finding of thieves, stolen property and murdered bodies. Of most relevance to this dissertation, of course, is the fact that there is now a substantial body of information about medical radiesthesia.[1]

## The mystical rod

As mentioned above, dowsing was known to most civilisations. The cradle lands of civilisation, the Indians of the two Americas, the Zulus, Maoris and the peoples of the far North and South, all of them have throughout time enjoyed the services of dowsers.

In Antiquity, dowsers mostly used some form of rod or wand. This can be seen from the pictures which have come down to us throughout the ages. From Egyptian tomb friezes to the paintings of the masters, the rod has been the major association with the dowser. Indeed, the traditional name for dowsing and water-divining was *rhabdomancy*, from the Greek *rhabdos*, meaning rod.

The fact that dowsing was probably regarded as the domain of the shaman or sorcerer-priest survives in the main attribute of the popular image of the witch, wizard and magician — the magic wand.

The 'rod' has been the standard tool for dowsing water, minerals and ores over the centuries. Indeed, its use is mentioned in various texts written by monks during the Dark Ages. In 1556, Georgius Agricola, a physician and the founding father of the science of mineralogy wrote a book entitled *De Re Metallica*. In it he discusses the use of the divining rod in searching for mineral veins. An illustration in the book even shows a dowser working with a forked hazel branch.

Perhaps as a result of that work the use of dowsers spread across Europe. The growth of the tin-mining industry in Cornwall, England, is even thought to owe much to the dowser's art. During the Elizabethan Age German miners were brought over and commissioned to dowse for tin veins.

Over the next century, however, dowsing by and large fell into disrepute. The Church considered it to be the work of the Devil. Indeed, the practice of dowsing could put an individual in peril of the Inquisition.

## The pendulum

It is to the Romans that most modern dowsers owe a debt. It was they who developed the *Art of Dactylomancy*, or pendulum dowsing. At the College of Augurs in Rome[2] they taught the use of swinging finger rings on fine threads in order to divine answers. Hence the term meant finger divination, from the word *dactulos*, meaning finger.

Although, as we have seen earlier, the rod has been the universal field-method for dowsing, the pendulum has many advantages for indoor work. It is probably true to say that it opens up a whole range of dowsing activities, which the rod is less well adapted to perform.

It was a professor of the medical faculty at Strasbourg, Gerboin, who 'invented' the dowser's pendulum in 1798. He conducted research on pendulum movements over different metals over a ten-year period, publishing in 1808.

Following Gerboin's work, the two famous scientists, Ampère[3] and Michel-Eugène Chevreul,[4] set out to determine whether the pendulum movements were controlled by sight and muscular movements. Neither were sensitive users themselves and came to negative conclusions. Chevreul concluded that the movements were all subconscious and not the result of radiation being picked up by the pendulum.

Other experimenters did not agree with Chevreul. One was F. de Briche, a former Secretary General of the Loiret, who constructed an ingenious apparatus in 1838. This consisted of an oak frame containing the pendulum. The only actual contact between the operator and the pendulum was by touching the thread with one finger. His belief was that this simple touch was all that was necessary in order to energise the pendulum to respond.

In 1851 Rutter of Brighton devised another experimental apparatus which he called the 'magnetoscope'. His aim was to isolate the pendulum from direct contact. The premise that he started with was that the movements of the pendulum came about through both animal and natural magnetism, both areas being fashionable at the time.

At this point Baron von Reichenbach entered the scene.[5] A scientific dilettante, he read about Rutter's work and travelled to Brighton to discuss the pendulum phenomenon. Returning home he himself devised numerous increasingly complicated pieces of apparatus in order to determine the nature of the pendulum activity.

He concluded: 'Bodies are surrounded by a sort of atmosphere, the effects of which can be ascertained, and measured, an atmosphere which the ordinary mortal cannot see, but which manifests itself by visible and concrete effects directly to it.'

Much of the early work this century was done in France. As mentioned above, it was the Abbé Alexis Bouley who introduced the term radiesthesia. Both he and another cleric, the Abbé Alexis Mermet, trained many radiesthetists in the art in the years after World War I.

Mermet in particular became greatly renowned and attracted clients from every corner of the world. His book, *Principles and Practice of Radiesthesia*, was to become the standard work on the subject. His major contribution was in introducing means of quantifying the pendulum's response, rather than merely relying upon qualitative results of the yes/no variety.

It was almost inevitable that radiesthesia would find much application in the field of health. Here the name of Dr Albert Abrams stands out. He can perhaps be said to be the father of medical radiesthesia and the related subject of radionics.[6] Dr Abrams used both a pendulum and an electrical apparatus for diagnosing health problems at a distance.

## Radionics

Shortly after World War I, Dr Albert Abrams discovered that when he was examining a patient with a cancer of the lip he could detect an area of dullness to percussion over the patient's abdomen. Incredibly, however, this only occurred when the patient was facing West! Dr Abrams concluded that this phenomenon had to be due to some radiational effect and interaction with the Earth's magnetic field.

Over the following years Abrams researched the subject of radiesthesia and developed an instrumentation method of measuring the radiation from different disease states. He developed and marketed a Black Box, which was capable of 'radiational diagnosis'. This instrument he called a *Reflexophone*.

Almost inevitably, the orthodox medical establishment scoffed at his discoveries and claims. Abrams became embittered and died a bitterly disappointed man.

In Britain a homoeopathic physician, Dr William Boyd, investigated Abrams' Black Box and devised his own machine, which he called an *Emanometer*. Although he was sceptical of many of Abrams' claims he also received very interesting results which convinced him that there was indeed something in this new subject of radionics — as the study of electrical instrumentation in radiesthesia had come to be called. In turn, his results were investigated by a committee set up under the direction of Lord Horder.

The results of the investigation were favourable, although the mechanism of action was concluded to be untraceable. The results were duly published in the *British Medical Journal* in 1924.

Research in radiesthesia continued in France. Turenne, an engineer and competent radiesthetist, was the first to produce prepared samples of various bodily organs. These *Turenne witnesses*[7] were to become standard tools in radiesthetic work.

Antoine Bovis was another interesting character who performed much research with the pendulum. Indeed, so strongly did he believe in his radiesthetic ability that he considered that scientific verification of his findings was unnecessary. His contributions have more relevance to radionics than to Psionic Medicine, yet his input was significant in the stimulus that he provided to later workers.

After Abrams died, his work was taken up in the USA by Ruth Drown, a chiropractor who had worked with him. She removed electrical circuitry from her machines, using only the body's natural energy to produce both diagnostic information and therapeutic intervention. It was this claim that the machines could actually 'broadcast' treatment that caused her problems.

In 1951, after two decades of successful and lucrative practice, she was arrested for fraud and medical quackery. An order was made that her instruments were to be destroyed. By the 1960s the use of radionics machines were banned and declared illegal in the USA. After a short period of imprisonment, she suffered two strokes and died in 1966.

Investigation in the Eastern Bloc countries and in the UK continued, however. George de la Warr, the most notable early radionics practitioner and researcher in Britain, developed a radionic camera apparently capable of photographing the energetic body from a blood spot.

In 1960, George de la Warr was also involved in a legal action. He was, however, cleared of all charges of fraud. Unfortunately, the judge stated that the scientific validity of the radionic method could not be accepted. While he was researching more radionic processes, George de la Warr died suddenly of a heart attack in 1965.

Malcolm Rae was the next major researcher in British radionics. Among his inventions were more sophisticated radionics machines and homoeopathic potentisers.

The works of the late Dr David Tansley,[8] a chiropractor, then took radionics to — *literally* — a higher plane, when he started analysing not only the physical body but also the subtle body of man.

### The birth of the psionic method[9]

In the 1930s Dr Guyon Richards, a homoeopath, was practising in London, using Abrams' techniques. At the outbreak of the war, however, his consulting room in London was bombed, destroying all of his radionic equipment. This led him to concentrate upon the use of the pendulum and the rule.[10]

Discovering other doctors exploring the same territory, Dr Richards was instrumental in forming the Medical Society for the Study of Radiesthesia (MSSR)[11] in 1939. He was the first Secretary and later President. Much of Guyon Richards' experiences were written down in his book, *The Chain of Life,* before he died in 1946.

One of the founding members of the MSSR was Dr George Laurence. After a broad and varied career he retired from general practice and devoted himself to the study of radiesthesia. In particular, he desired to find out what were the basic causes of illness and disease.

Laurence had been strongly influenced by the earlier work of McDonagh and his Unitary Theory of Disease (see Chapter Seven). He found that by using his radiesthetic faculty he was able to corroborate the concept that diseases are mainly functions of protein imbalance or aberration, and that cure can only be achieved if that aberration is restored.

He was also drawn by Hahnemann's Miasmic Theory of Chronic Disease. He found that the detection, recognition and elimination of miasms were necessary in the treatment of chronic disease and for future prevention. Going further than that, however, he became aware of acquired miasms, or as he termed them *'retained toxins of acquired infections'.* (This has of course been extended further to include many more infections, metals, radiations, etc — see Chapter Six on Miasms and Toxins, by Dr Farley Spink.)

Homoeopathy was the treatment modality which Laurence found ideally suited to correct the protein imbalances. He believed that they worked by virtue of the specific 'vital essence' — *Vis Medicatrix* — of each remedy which allowed it to work at the supersensible level needed by the patient.

The works of Rudolf Steiner[12] proved the final basis for

Laurence. In particular, he drew on Steiner's concept of the four-fold make-up of Man — the physical, etheric, astral bodies, and the ego. The concept of the Vital Force, as advocated by Hahnemann, was reaffirmed and became central to his thought.

Dr Aubrey T. Westlake had also joined the MSSR in 1942 and had conducted much research himself. He and Laurence were to be associated for many years. Indeed, in 1964 Westlake visited Laurence in order to record the methods of diagnosis and treatment that he had devised. This was subsequently published in *Practical Dowsing* in 1965 under the title 'The Laurence Technique of Psionic Diagnosis and Treatment'.

A fundamental aspect of this was the use of the Triangle chart — the *Laurence chart* — which, as Westlake says: 'provides a means of determining an equilibrium of forces radiesthetically between three factors — the patient's blood spot, the disease witness (usually a Turenne) and the indicated homoeopathic or other remedy. So here we have a firm basis for the practical application of Psionic Medicine, and it has also proved suitable for instruction and teaching.'

By 1968 there had been sufficient further research and increased interest shown in order to form the Psionic Medical Society. The membership consisted of qualified doctors and dentists, and lay associates and supporters. At that time there were over 120 members. Dr George Laurence was elected President, Dr Aubrey Westlake Vice-President and Mr Carl Upton the first Secretary.

In 1975 the Institute of Psionic Medicine was founded with the aim of providing teaching instruction and ongoing support for qualified doctors and dentists. Mr Carl Upton was the first Secretary and Dr Gordon Flint the first Dean.

## The Psionic Medical Society and the Institute of Psionic Medicine

The Psionic Medical Society, as mentioned above, was formed in 1968. It is a registered charity, set up to promote the wider application of the system. Membership is open to patients, practitioners and people who are genuinely interested in the system. An annual meeting takes place in order that Society members might meet practitioners and other interested individuals, and learn more about the subject from invited speakers. It publishes occasional papers and the annual *Journal of the Psionic Medical Society & the Institute of Psionic Medicine (JPMS&IPM)*.

The Institute of Psionic Medicine is the professional body, which is responsible for research and training in the methods of Psionic Medicine. At this moment in time Membership and Fellowship is **only** available to qualified doctors, dentists and veterinary surgeons, all of whom have to pass through a recognised training scheme.

At the time of writing, three prerequisites are ordinarily considered to be necessary prior to training:

1. A medical, dental or veterinary qualification, registerable in the UK (or its equivalent abroad).
2. A working background knowledge of homoeopathy.
3. The ability to dowse. Competence in the use of the pendulum is essential and the British Society of Dowsers has undertaken to train interested doctors, dentists and veterinary surgeons prior to their introduction to the medical applications.

Thereafter, training requires that the candidate should attend the Institute of Psionic Medicine, being assigned to a personal tutor who will instruct the student in the use of charts, samples and witnesses. After a period of time, the student will move on to the diagnosis of cases and, after demonstrating competence in psionic analysis, start to treat patients (again under personal supervision).

There is a minimum time of tuition, but no maximum, the very nature of psionic analysis being such that people take different lengths of time in order to develop the necessary skill. After treating no less than 100 cases (under supervision of the tutor), the candidate is then expected to submit to the examining board a dissertation of original research within the field, then take an examination covering all subjects within the Psionic Medicine curriculum. Upon satisfactory completion of training and success in the dissertation and the examination, the qualification of Member of the Institute of Psionic Medicine (MIPsiMed) may be conferred upon the candidate.

[1]At this point I am still going to use the term medical radiesthesia, since it was not until the work of George Laurence that the term Psionic Medicine was used. Apparently he first coined the term in 1962.

[2]The Emperor Claudius (Tiberius Claudius Drusus Nero Germanicus 10BC to 54AD), nephew of Tiberius, uncle of Caligula, the conqueror of Britain in 43AD, was an appointed augur.

Augurs were respected Roman officials (the College of Augurs originally consisted of three patricians, extended by the Ogulnian law of 300BC to include five plebians and four patricians, then later to 15 — appointments granted for life). Their function was to read omens and portents from which auspices could be taken. They read the weather, the flight of birds, the feeding of the sacred chickens, the behaviour of four-footed animals and the movement of finger rings — dactylomancy.

They were readers of trends, not foretellers of the future or of fortune.

[3]André Marie Ampère (1775–1836), French physicist who propounded the theory that magnetism is the result of molecular electric currents. The unit of electrical current, the Ampere or Amp, is named after him.

[4]Chevreul used an iron ring suspended from thread as his standard pendulum.

[5]Baron Karl von Reichenbach, German physicist, was born at Stuttgart; acquired considerable property by foundries which he established in Moravia. He discovered paraffin and creosote, and maintained the existence of the imponderable agent, which he called Od, and which he supposed to be distributed throughout nature — see later text.

Among his chief works were: *Geological Researches in Moravia* (1834), *Researches on Magnetism* (1842), *Odische-Magnetische Briefe* (1852).

[6]Radionics is the name given to the use of electronic apparatus combined with the radiesthetic faculty in order to arrive at a diagnosis and to broadcast a treatment to the patient.

[7]Turenne witnesses were supplied in boxes of 40, consisting of starch-impregnated powder in small glass vials. Turenne witnesses representing the various diseases to which man is prone were also available — see Vernon D. Wethered's book *The Practice of Medical Radiesthesia*, (C.W. Daniels).

Nowadays, witnesses are prepared in homoeopathic doses, usually a single tablet or a quantity of granules to a vial. The potency is normally 12c, although it is often necessary to use other potencies when looking at different energetic levels.

[8]The late David Tansley, a chiropractor and radionics practitioner, wrote a series of books in the 1970s and 1980s which revolutionised radionic thinking. Heavily influenced by eastern philosophy and the esoteric works of Alice A. Bailey they make fascinating, if complicated, reading.

[9]This section is drawn from the book *Psionic Medicine* by Reyner, Laurence and Upton, Routledge & Kegan Paul, 1974, second edition 1982, and from the article *The Origins and History of Psionic Medicine* by Aubrey T. Westlake, reproduced from a lecture given at a weekend conference of the Institute of Psionic Medicine, June 1977.

[10]The rule was the commonest radiesthetic tool used in early practice. Guyon Richards used a 48-inch rule — in actual fact the 48-inch edge of his desk!

[11]The Medical Society for the Study of Radiesthesia lasted from 1939 until 1975. In 1942, when Dr Aubrey Westlake joined, there were 34 medical members and 15 associates (only medically qualified individuals were eligible for full membership).

[12]Rudolf Steiner (1861–1925) was a German educationalist and mystic. Originally an adherent of Madame Blavatsky's Theosophical Movement, he broke away in 1913 to form his own '*Anthroposophical Society*'.

Steiner's works have had an influence on very many areas of intellectual thought — education, architecture, art and of course medicine.

# Practical Dowsing

*'Practice, that excellent master, has taught me many things.'*

**Pliny the Younger (AD62–113)**

owsing with a pendulum is an ancient art, but its systematic application — radiesthesia — as an aid to scientific research or to medical diagnosis, as seen in the last chapter, is comparatively new.

There is no special power in the pendulum as such. It is simply a convenient instrumental aid, of which the value depends entirely upon the sensitivity of the dowsing faculty of the operator. If this were not so, then the pendulum would react irrespective of the physical contact with the dowser.

A pendulum is, in fact, a simple means of magnifying and rendering visible certain impulses of a biodynamic character that are activated in the dowser by his paranormal senses. Effectively this movement is an *ideomotor response*, or an unconscious muscular reaction.[1]

The pendulum itself, as the name suggests, consists of a weight or bob suspended by thread or fine chain. It can take any form, provided it can be held comfortably by the operator and swing freely above the particular 'field' to be examined.

A length of about 10cm is convenient while a bob may be of any material such as crystal, glass, plastic or wood. Metal may be used, though it is thought preferable to use some inert material.

The weight is a matter of personal preference. A light bob will provide a rapid response but may be influenced by air currents or unsteadiness of the hand, while a heavy bob may be sluggish in its response. A weight of about 10g is convenient.

The shape of the bob is again a matter of personal choice, although a shaped or pointed end acts as a natural pointer. A spherical bob may be confusing when working with charts (which we shall touch on later in this chapter), but attaching a short length of chain to the base of the bob will give a clearer indication.

## Pendulum movements

There are three basic movements, namely:

1. A simple to-and-fro oscillation usually, but not necessarily, towards and away from the operator.
2. A rotary motion in a clockwise direction.
3. A similar rotary movement anticlockwise.

It is these movements or combinations thereof, which provide the answers to the questions being posed; but there is no hard and fast rule. Everyone has to find, by individual experiment, how to interpret these movements. A particular reaction that may indicate to one dowser a certain situation may, to another, suggest the opposite, so that one has to establish by trial one's individual pattern, which with practice will be found to be consistent.

## Mental questioning

Before putting the pendulum into operation the dowser must have clearly in mind the question it is desired to elucidate. The question must be direct and expressed in the simplest terms possible. Any ambiguity is bound to result in ambiguous and inconclusive results. It is an axiom in dowsing that nonsense begets nonsense.

When formulating a question to which an answer is required there must be no prejudice in the mind of the dowser. Any mental preconceptions or suggestions, which occupy the mind of the operator, are bound to confuse the dowsing faculty and the indications of the pendulum will be worthless. It is for this reason that 'arranged' tests to satisfy curiosity, to convince sceptics, or merely tricks and showmanship should be avoided at all costs. No serious dowser tolerates such impositions since anything outside the pure and simple questions with which the enquiry is concerned will nullify the findings and makes the operation valueless. Such superimposition is inevitable in the circumstances named.

## Obtaining dowsing responses

The first requirement is to develop the facility for oneself, for which purpose we may commence with a few simple experiments. Sit comfortably at a table on which there is a sheet of white paper, such as a paper tissue. Place on this a pencil or pen and hold the pendulum lightly between the thumb and the first (or second) finger over the middle of the object. The hand and arm should be quite relaxed, and it is helpful at the beginning to rest the elbow on the table to keep the hand steady. One should, in fact, be relaxed in body and mind, the mental relaxation being initially the more difficult. One must not expect any particular reaction, but at the same time one must be ready for a response, for if one believes nothing will happen, this very attitude will inhibit any reaction.

After a short time the pendulum will start to oscillate along the length of the pencil. Allow the oscillation to build up to a reasonable swing and then gently move the hand towards the tip of the pencil where the motion will slowly change to a rotation. If the hand is now moved slowly towards the other end of the pencil the pendulum will revert to the oscillating mode until it reaches the other end, where it will rotate, this time in the opposite direction.

At first the pendulum may take a little time to respond. Begin with a length of about 10cm, but if it is unduly reluctant to start, try altering the length slightly either way. By experiment one soon finds the length best suited to one's personal requirements and with practice it will be found to start swinging almost immediately. However, if there is still no response, wait and try later; one is probably not sufficiently relaxed. In any case, make the attempt alone, for until one has developed the ability, the presence of others is distracting.

One need not be concerned with the reason for this behaviour, for the object of the exercise is merely the acquisition of the basic expertise. In simple terms, any physical object is a local condensation of the etheric field, which can be regarded as flowing through the object. With this, the pendulum tends to align itself but, at the extremities, the field is no longer confined and begins to spread out in all directions, so that the pendulum goes into a gyratory motion. Some exponents of the art pursue this field distribution in detail, but for the present purposes this is neither necessary nor desirable. The pendulum is, in fact, simply answering the mental question, *Is there an object here?*

Even when a response is obtained, do not continue the experiment for more than a brief period, because this creates a tendency to *will* the behaviour of the pendulum, which is very easily done, and can produce spurious indications. It is the initial unconscious reactions that are genuine, and the experiment should be only of brief duration, but repeated at frequent intervals until the reactions occur with increasingly short delays as the facility develops.

A further reason for not prolonging the test is that there is an inherent tendency for the rhythm to change. For example, if the pendulum is gyrating over a sample it will after a certain time change to an oscillation and after a similar period will revert to gyration in the opposite direction. The number of swings in each mode depends upon the substance under examination, and this is utilised by some dowsers to obtain specific information. For the present purpose this is not required and may be ignored, but it is clear that it could confuse the beginner if the test is continued for too long.

Another pitfall of which the beginner must be wary is repetition. Finding himself in some doubt about a reading he may be inclined to repeat the procedure, possibly several times. This is to be avoided since it tends to induce a state of mind confusing to the dowsing faculty. The first readings are the most reliable if the mind is clear and the question precise. If there is an overall inconsistency or lack of clarity, all readings should be suspect and it is better to defer further work until mental and other conditions are more favourable.

## Posing questions

One can now begin to use the pendulum to answer simple questions. Hold the pendulum over a copper coin of any convenient denomination (or currency) and allow it to build up a gyration. With the free hand touch a second (similar) coin as a *witness*[2] and observe what happens. Then repeat the experiment with a different witness — e.g., a piece of steel, such as a penknife, or a sample of (genuine) silver, and again observe the reaction.

After a little practice it will be found that in the first case the pendulum will cease to gyrate and will begin to swing to and fro towards the witness, but in the second case it will not alter its mode. This is actually a response to an unconscious enquiry, *Are these two objects of similar material?* — Of course, one knows this to be the case with the two identical coins; with a witness of different material there is no affinity and the pendulum will not change its mode, indicating the answer, *No*.

However, if the experiment is now repeated using a modern socalled silver coin as a witness — e.g., a five-pence piece or a dime — the pendulum will again swing towards the witness, suggesting that the coins are of identical material, which they clearly are not. This is a significant example of loose questioning, for in fact both coins contain a predominance of copper and to this extent are of similar constitution; but if one asks mentally, *Are these coins of **identical** composition?* the pendulum will not deviate, giving a clear answer, *No*.

So, learn to be specific and unambiguous in your mental questioning. Actually formulate the question in words in your mind.

## Water divining

Water divining is an important and well-known aspect of dowsing and it provides a useful source of experience for the aspirant to medical dowsing. Perhaps the simplest test is to hold the pendulum over a glass of water and, after starting an oscillation, to watch its subsequent behaviour. As a variant of this exercise the pendulum can first be held a little to one side of the glass and then moved over the glass to the opposite side, noting any change of swing during the process.

Once a consistent reaction has been obtained to the presence of water, further tests can be made over a known water pipe or stream to develop further familiarity with the behaviour of the pendulum. It is then only a short step to water divining proper in its elementary application, namely the location of a hidden underground well or stream, or other location where water is situated.

It will sometimes be noticed that the pendulum gives no response on commencing to dowse. This may occur for a number of reasons, but one of the commonest is connected with the distance the pendulum is held away from the object of study. When beginning to dowse, move the pendulum slowly up or down, increasing or decreasing the distance from the object until a response is achieved.

This is a valuable exercise because under different conditions of speed of flow, depth, or chemical or bacterial content the pendulum will reflect differences in intensity and speed of swing which can eventually become valuable indicators in medical work.

## Dowsing over living tissue

We come now to a whole series of possibilities for the beginner who has gained some familiarity with the pendulum and its behaviour. We can begin to observe how the pendulum reacts to living tissue.

Hold the pendulum over the back of a lightly clenched fist and observe the swing. Now do the same over the hand of someone of the opposite sex.

Having absorbed the lesson of this simple exercise, smack the back of the hand smartly and watch the reaction of the pendulum again. Repeat the check over the course of half an hour or so and observe any changes in pendulum behaviour that might occur.

Then one may extend the enquiry by watching the reaction of the pendulum to various parts of the body. It will be found probably that not only are there variations in swing in different parts, but also between healthy and unhealthy tissue and organs. But, of course, considerable experience is necessary to be able to interpret such data.

It is very useful to be able to check the vitality of objects that occur in nature. By holding the pendulum above the object under test one can note the type and character of swing and can deduce information of great value. But, here again, it is important to frame specific questions with precision.

It is possible to make qualitative evaluations of all manner of material. In the simple testing of a packet of garden seeds before planting, or of some fruit or vegetable before eating, one has a most fascinating and useful yardstick to vitality. In these days of devitalised foods this test can become a significant health aid.

Whether a particular item of food is good for one personally or not can be put to the test. One method, with the question in mind, is to swing the pendulum for a few moments over the back of the hand to get a characteristic reaction and then slowly move the hand over the food. Any change in swing will indicate whether the food in question is either indifferent or definitely harmful, according to one's personal pendulum convention. Another method is merely to point the index finger of the free hand towards the article to be tested and observe the swing, having of course posed the necessary question.

Poisonous substances may be checked in this way too, but it is not advisable to rely upon such a test unless one has considerable experience as a medical dowser.

## Introducing measurement

So far we have been concerned with exercises intended to familiarise the beginner with typical pendulum responses or with straightforward yes or no questions. But in medical dowsing, and particularly in the techniques of Psionic Medicine, quantitative indications are required. Comparative diagnosis, degree and location of involvement of disease processes and their cause now take place in the dowser's experience.

The pendulum will be called upon to work with two or more witnesses. Devices for recording measurements of degree of pendulum deviation from a point of balance or norm must be introduced. The most usual of these are rules for linear measurements and charts indicating angular deviations.

Two such aids will be considered. The first is the rule, which is simple to produce. Take a strip of wood 100cm long and mark it out in 1cm intervals, numbered 50–0–50. Mark the left hand +50 and the right hand –50 (Figure 10). Exercises may then be tried by placing witnesses on the extreme right or left ends (over the 50) and swinging the pendulum to and fro across the rule. The swing will normally be horizontal, but as the pendulum is moved along the rule a point will be found where the swing changes to a vertical movement across the rule. This is called the balance point from which the desired information may be deduced.

You may begin by placing a sample of your own hair on the –50 point. Start by dowsing over the hair, then begin moving the dowsing hand along the rule. Note where the balance point is reached. And get into the habit of asking a specific question each time, e.g., *Where is my personal balance point?*

Next put a small sample of food at the zero and repeat the process, again starting from the hair sample. Ask the question,

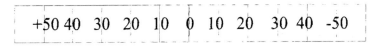

+50 40  30  20  10   0  10  20   30  40  -50

*Figure 10*

*What effect will this food have on me?* If the food is beneficial to you, the balance point will be in the positive range. If it is neutral it will make no difference to the personal balance point you achieved only with your hair. If it is bad for you (either sensitivity or possibly allergy) you will get a negative reading. Alternatively, place the food sample at the +50 with the hair again at –50 and dowse over each in turn; this helps you to 'pick up' or focus on the two witnesses. Then dowse along the rule to get the balance point of the hair (you) and the food. The position of the balance point in negative or positive will tell you about how the food is for you.

This basic testing can be repeated for drugs, various metals and homoeopathic remedies. An excellent beginner's lesson is also to be found in testing the Bach Flower Remedies.[3] It is easy to find out which of these remedies are good for oneself, or others, but seeing how the selection of the right remedy may vary according to their state of mind (jealousy, anger, impatience, etc), is highly instructive.

The next aid is the circle and triangle chart used in the Laurence-Upton technique of Psionic Medicine. This chart consists of a circle within a triangle, as illustrated in Figure 11. The radius of the circle is 5cm; the long side of the triangle being 30cm; while from the centre of the circle a series of radial lines is drawn at ten-degree intervals.

Having constructed such a figure on white paper or card, various exercises can be tried. First place a two-pence coin in the right hand angle of the triangle and in the left a piece of copper wire. Swing the pendulum over the centre of the circle in a to-and-fro motion along the vertical line running through the apex of the triangle and then allow it to take its own course. Observe the degree of any deviation to right or left. Then reverse the positions of the coin and copper wire, coin on the left and wire on the right. Once again observe the deviation.

Then repeat the exercises with a sample of your hair, placed in the right-hand corner of the triangle and a sample of food in the left. Also, try testing out homoeopathic remedies, or Bach Flower

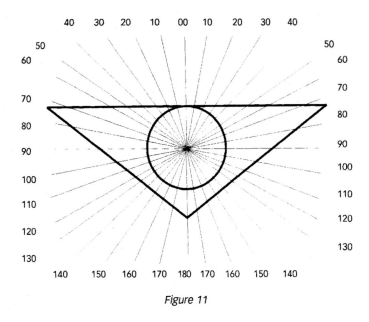

*Figure 11*

Remedies, by placing them in the left-hand corner and record your results. Remember, however, to have a clear question framed in your mind as you do so. The effect of placing a third object or substance near the apex of the triangle can also be tried.

It is emphasised that these exercises are intended only as a convenient way of getting used to the pendulum in conjunction with a chart. The principle, however, is fundamental to the diagnostic techniques used in Psionic Medicine.

These various exercises will serve to introduce the aspirant to the art of dowsing in order to develop a certain facility with the pendulum. The student should record his (or her) reactions with a view to establishing a coherent pattern of response. He can then begin to devise for himself various extensions and modifications to increase his experience, and try to co-ordinate his conclusions.

At this stage it becomes possible to develop the faculty more precisely, but for this, particularly in any attempts at medical dowsing, it is necessary to seek expert instruction.

[1] In radionic testing, the unconscious perception seems to be transmitted through the autonomic nervous system. In radiesthesia, the central nervous system seems to be stimulated, resulting in the unconscious ideomotor response.

[2] A witness is the name given to a sample of a known material, or a specific specimen (often in homoeopathic potency) of a remedy, organ or tissue. These are usually kept in separate vials for ready usage with psionic charts.

[3] The full set of 38 remedies covers most of the negative emotional states which one is liable to come across. Most people have about five or six recurrent negative states, so finding out which remedies are appropriate for them can make life very much more bearable.

# The Psionic Approach

*Tolle Causam* (Seek the Cause)

**The motto of the Psionic Medical Society**

The above motto sums up the aim of Psionic Medicine. Rather than merely aiming at relieving symptoms of illness, the psionic practitioner is striving to find the underlying cause of the problem. This goes much deeper than the usual search performed in orthodox medicine, where the aim of diagnosis is to reach a diagnostic label. Rather than being satisfied with merely diagnosing someone as having Rheumatoid Arthritis, for example, a psionic approach would try find the cause of the disturbance within the personal psi-field that has led to bio-chemical, functional and structural alterations in the immune and musculoskeletal systems, resulting in the symptom cluster which is diagnosed as Rheumatoid Arthritis. Having ascertained the cause and nature of the imbalances, the next step is to define the best treatment. In most cases the mainstay of treatment will be some form of homoeopathic medication, usually supported by dietary or other appropriate advice.

The basic method used (and taught) by the Institute of Psionic Medicine is the *Laurence-Upton technique of analysis*. As we shall see, this utilises a pendulum, the Laurence-Upton chart, a specimen from the patient and a set of witnesses.

## Disturbances in the personal psi-field

The personal psi-field is both *informational* and *organisational*. It contains the entire history of all that has happened to the individual, whose essence we may term the soul. And as we saw in Chapter Four on the Subtle Bodies, it contains the thought and emotional fields and the etheric body. At deep levels it connects with the collective unconsciousness, the species morphogenetic field, and is possibly influenced by karmic and acquisition fields. Also, it interacts with the physical body through various subtle mechanisms (chakric and meridian systems and the direct etheric–physical interface), and it interacts with the body's proteins. This we represent as a personal ray, or beam (see Figure 7, Chapter Four).

The *informational* aspect of the field contains:
- Access to the collective unconscious with its symbolism and archetypes
- The information common to the species
- Possibly karmic information
- Acquired characteristics, both inherited and personal
- Emotions
- Mind — consciousness and personal unconscious

The *organisational* aspect of the field consists of :
- Chakric system
- Meridian system
- Direct etheric–physical interface
- Mind — consciousness, and personal unconscious

These exert a controlling and organisational effect upon the physical body whereby:
- Mind and emotional fields can affect the physical body, via psychoneuroimmunological routes
- Cellular biochemistry is affected
- Tissue, organ and system function is affected
- Physical structure undergoes pathological change

Effectively, it can produce a trickle down effect through our model of the pyramid of medicine (Figure 12).

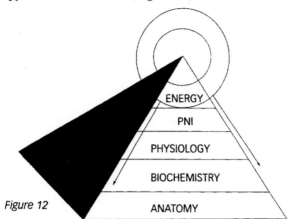

Figure 12

At this point it helps to conceptualise the personal psi-field as a sphere, rather than a ray. Within the field, like the layers of an onion, or perhaps more appropriately like the layers of a pearl, every experience, trauma, miasm and toxin is recorded. *(Understand that within the field these are not in layers as such, this is merely a three-dimensional explanatory model.)*

As the individual's self-regulating mechanisms (their 'mind', immune and homoeostatic mechanisms) cope with each of these, they are effectively 'walled off', or inactivated. They are seemingly relegated to the past. In reality, however, the *'event'* (be it experience, trauma, miasm or toxin) continues to exert an effect, in that it contributes to the overall dynamic nature of the individual. In terms of our model, think of the whole field as having a composite vibration. And think of any *event* as having a particular *'vibration'*, or *'perturbation'*. The less of a problem it is, the smaller the vibration, so the less of an effect it has on the overall psi-field 'vibration'.

Some of these layers may be harder to deal with than others. Because they may 'vibrate' out of phase with the field they may cause a taint on the smooth-functioning of the psi-field, indeed completely affecting the way it operates and organises the physical body. It may only be held in check, prevented from agitating, by the energy within the next layers, which is effectively operating as a containment layer. But if it becomes active, starts to vibrate out of phase, then its effects (which can be either stimulatory or inhibitory in a functional sense) can be manifest throughout the whole of the field, *to affect the etheric body, emotional field and thought field.* This will reduce the overall *vitality* of the field. These effects are then conveyed to the physical body by the subtle connections, so that a perception of being unwell is experienced.

Let us consider a few examples:

1. *High vitality with no perturbation* (Figure 13). In this situation, the individual has high vitality and the miasms and toxins are causing no problem. The psi-field is 'balanced', so the subtle connections function well and the individual perceives himself to feel well.

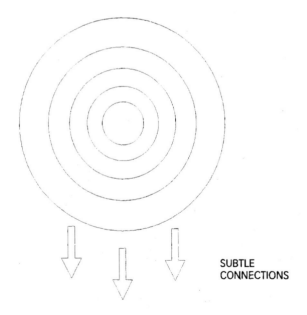

SUBTLE
CONNECTIONS

FEELS WELL                                   *Figure 13*

2. *Moderate vitality with slight perturbation* (Figure 14). In this situation the vitality is reduced because of a deep-seated agitating miasm. It produces a niggling chronic condition. An example would be a tubercular miasm producing a problem like insomnia or migraine.

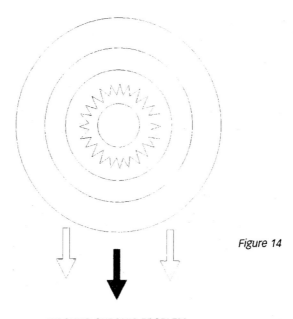

Figure 14

NIGGLING CHRONIC PROBLEM

3. *Moderate vitality with slight perturbation and lowered resistance* (Figure 15). In this situation an agitating toxin, such as an acquired aluminium toxin, is producing a perturbation which is just being kept under control and contained by another event layer. A new problem, such as a bowel infection or gastric flu, causes a lowering of resistance which weakens the containment layer, allowing the agitating aluminium toxin to cause a major perturbation. This could result in an irritable bowel problem or a more serious inflammatory bowel disease.

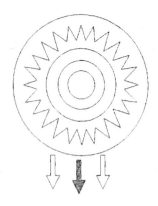

ALUMINIUM LAYER
NIGGLING BUT CONTAINED

ONLY SLIGHT PROBLEMS

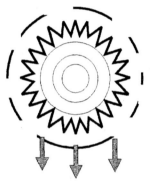

NEW INFECTION LOWERS RESISTANCE

ALUMINIUM LAYER NOT WELL
CONTAINED

PROBLEMS WORSEN

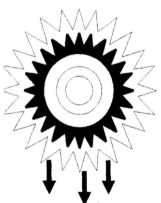

ALUMINIUM LAYER OVERCOMES
CONTAINMENT LAYER

MAJOR PERTURBATION

WORSENING SYMPTOMS
WITH SERIOUS POTENTIAL

*Figure 15*

4. *Lowered vitality due to suppressant treatment* (Figure 16) . This is often seen in the classic problem with eczema and asthma. When the eczema is treated with suppressant therapy (such as steroid creams), there is an apparent dispersal effect or improvement of the skin. However, this is often followed after a 'honeymoon phase' by a flare-up of the asthma. This happens because the toxins causing the asthma are no longer contained, because the suppression has weakened the containment. This situation is seen with many suppressant treatments. Patients may feel that it is as if the treatment has driven the condition internally only for it to manifest in another form.

INACTIVE TOXINS ASSOCIATED
WITH:

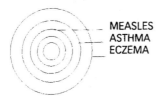 MEASLES
ASTHMA
ECZEMA

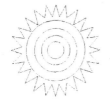 ACTIVE ECZEMA

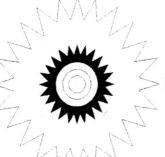 APPARENT ECZEMA DISPERSAL
FOLLOWED BY ASTHMA FLARE-UP

*Figure 16*

Antibiotic treatment is, of course, a powerful suppressant treatment, for the antibiotics act upon the bacteria which one carries within one. An article in a recent issue of the *British Medical Journal* (*BMJ*) commented that only 10 per cent of the cells in the human body mass are actually of human origin. In the context of the psi-field, this means that many millions of microbes, together with their psi-fields, are incorporated into the personal psi-field of the individual. Killing off a proportion of those microbes is bound to have a significant effect on the individual psi-field. Antibiotics are not, therefore, simple drugs to be taken ad hoc. Their use must be clearly indicated, for their effects are far-reaching.

5. *Lowered vitality with several layers agitating each other to produce a moderate or major perturbation* (Figure 17). In this

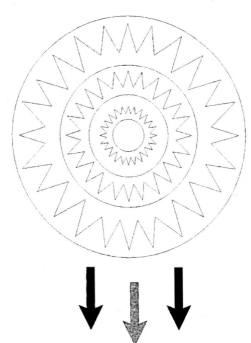

Figure 17

SEVERAL LAYERS AGITATING ONLY JUST BEING CONTAINED
SO MODERATE OR MAJOR PERTURBATION LIKELY

situation many things can happen, depending upon which toxins are present and on what area of the individual they are targetting. It can result in degenerative conditions, auto-immune disorders or severe emotional or psychological problems. This can happen if a syphilitic toxin is present, which may have a tendency to allow others to become agitated.

6. *Low vitality and chain reaction* (Figure 18). In this situation a deep toxin can start to agitate. And some seem to do so spontaneously

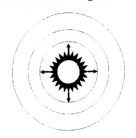

DEEP TOXIN CAUSING OUTWARD AGITATION

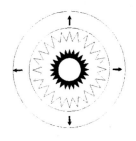

CONTAINMENT LAYER AGITATES, PRODUCING NEW SYMPTOMS

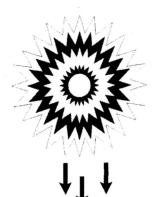

CHAIN REACTION.
MAJOR PERTURBATION RESULTS

*Figure 18*

at different times of life, presumably related to the vitality of the individual at that time in their life. This perturbation may be so powerful that it overcomes outer containment layers, causing them to agitate, to produce their own symptoms and illness. This layer can then affect the next and so on in a sort of chain reaction, until there is complete flare-up, and many things seem to go wrong in quick succession. This may occur when a deep miasm like gonorrhoea becomes active.

7. *Low vitality and triggering illness resulting in shut-down* (Figure 19). This situation can occur when a succession of toxins or miasms have been niggling away, producing a moderate perturbation, but the individual copes. Then a triggering illness causes a lowering of the containment layer, which was holding everything in check, so that the major flare-up results. The effect is so severe that the field almost goes into shut-down, using up all available vital energy to contain the problem. Multiple blocks occur in the subtle connections and the individual is left in a state of utter depletion. This is a possible mechanism in Chronic Fatigue Syndrome.

These mechanisms are merely put forward as models to illustrate the manner in which perturbations, or taints in the personal psi-field may become manifest as illness. It must be emphasised that there is no standard mechanism by which a person becomes ill. Each person is unique and each person's health and illness is unique to them.

Also, although we are talking about 'layers', these are only used as a model to facilitate understanding. The layers as such do not exist in a three-dimensional sense, but possibly exist as 'interference patterns' within the holographic nature of the field.

## The Laurence-Upton technique

As the reader is already well aware, Psionic Medicine uses the radiesthetic or dowsing faculty in order to tune into the individual's personal psi-field. This is done by focussing attention with

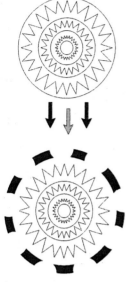

SEVERAL LAYERS AGITATING,
ONLY JUST BEING CONTAINED
SO MODERATE OR MAJOR
PERTURBATION LIKELY

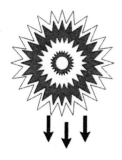

TRIGGERING ILLNESS WEAKENS
CONTAINMENT LAYER

MAJOR FLARE-UP

TOTAL SHUT-DOWN

SUBTLE CONNECTIONS BLOCKED

*Figure 19*

the pendulum upon a sample of the individual's hair or blood, effectively over a sample of their protein. This protein, although it is no longer physically connected with the individual, is still a part of their personal psi-field. Thus, it is able to furnish us with energetic information at that moment in time (see the sections on Interconnectedness in Chapters One and Four).

The actual technique was first developed by George Laurence, then jointly updated with Carl Upton, hence the name — the Laurence-Upton technique.

Both men felt strongly about how it should be practised and how it should be taught, so it is appropriate to let Carl Upton air his views:

'The techniques of Psionic Medicine involve on the one hand detailed knowledge and experience in the orthodox medical field, and on the other the ability to dowse in relation to samples and appropriates witnesses with the aid of suitable geometric patterns or rules to introduce the possibility of measurement in the evaluation of results.

'Essentially, the technique requires the mental formulation of specific questions arising out of the known clinical data related to the patient's medical history and current complaints. To such questions the response to the trained practitioner comes in the form of reactions indicated by the hand-held pendulum which is used to measure deviations from the norm, by reference to an appropriate chart. A knowledge of anatomy, physiology, pathology, bacteriology, pharmacology and practical experience in these subjects is a basic requirement; in addition to which the principles of medicine and surgery and familiarity with the elements of psychology are needed to enable the practitioner to frame in his mind the necessary formulation to convey to the dowsing faculty. A set of co-ordinates, as it were, must first be established and this depends upon the experience of the practitioner. Then the dowsing faculty is enabled to respond in meaningful terms, which can be understood in relation to the observed clinical data and history.

'Whereas in orthodox medical diagnostic procedure use is made of inference and standardised references either in the intellectual memory or in reference libraries, the logical conclusions being therefore indirect, in psionic medical techniques the conclusions reached are immediate and direct and stem from another dimension of knowledge.

'Where, as in orthodox diagnostic procedures, standardised references are used it is not difficult to set down definite rules of procedure. But where individual sensitivity is involved as a means towards diagnosis it is not possible to represent this adequately in any text. Indeed, any attempt to do so could lead to many misleading notions and consequent distortions, which could well prejudice the welfare of the patient and the reputation of the practitioner. It is for this reason that the techniques of Psionic Medicine can only be taught verbally and in person by an experienced practitioner.

'To enable any interested medical, dental or veterinary practitioner to gain some familiarity in a preparatory way with the pendulum the simple exercises in Chapter Ten are recommended. But the application of any facility thereby gained can only be related to the specific psionic medical techniques of diagnosis and remedy selection through personal instruction. It should perhaps be emphasised that until the candidate is able to use the pendulum successfully the techniques of Psionic Medicine cannot be taught. Equally, a pendulist who does not have the necessary basic medical knowledge and experience cannot be taught either.'

The restriction on training in the Laurence-Upton technique is actually written into the constitution of the Institute of Psionic Medicine. It is there as a safeguard for the public, not for any reason of nepotism.

The thing is that the process is not at all easy. One could liken it to fishing through a hole in the ice (Figure 20). Just as the fisherman may receive many sensations on his line, indicating tiny nibbles or big bites, from fish of many sizes, occurring at different depths, so may the pendulum indicate a whole range of possibilities. The skill is in being able to ask well-formulated, penetrating questions. This is why a thorough medical, dental or veterinary background is considered essential.

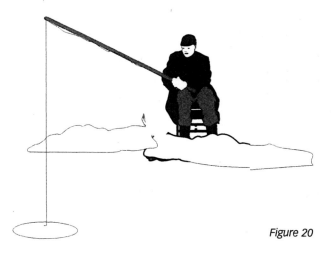

*Figure 20*

So, because it is considered necessary to teach by personal instruction, it is only possible to describe the technique in broad terms from now on. Yet having said that, we can usefully cover many of the principles involved so that the reader can get a fairly good idea of what is done.

### The Laurence-Upton chart, samples and witnesses
A description was given of this in Chapter Ten. By convention, the readings on the right-hand side of the chart are considered negative, while the left side is considered positive (Figure 21).

The patient sample (usually a blood specimen or a hair sample) is usually positioned in the right-hand angle of the triangle, while witnesses[1] of various sorts are placed in the left-hand angle. A standard psionic diagnostic set will have at least 200 separate witnesses of DNA, RNA, cells and cellular material, tissues, organs, systems, pathological specimens, microorgansisms, parasites, animal, vegetable and mineral poisons, etc. Having dowsed over each angle, to 'catch' their effect, the pendulum is then

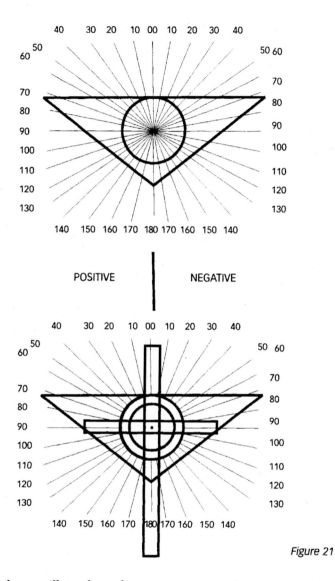

*Figure 21*

allowed to oscillate along the zero axis, any subsequent angular deviation being recorded.

Various cards allow a systematic approach to be used in order to facilitate the diagnostic process and to indicate which witnesses should be used.

Eventually, a totality reading of the imbalance of forces will be obtained along the horizontal axis (of a Celtic Cross pattern) which invites reconciliation (or rebalancing) through the introduction of appropriate force (the remedies) at the foot of the vertical axis.

## The creative triad

Special mention should be made of three witnesses, these being protein or amino acids, DNA and RNA. And again, it is perhaps appropriate to have Carl Upton's view on their significance:

'*DNA is ascribed the function as the carrier of genetic information. Protein is the fundamental material of which the tissues of the body are made and RNA is the catalyst that unites the two into a living whole. Hence, in terms of the creative triad, it would seem that DNA provides the expression of the form, protein gives substance to the genetic pattern, while RNA is the vehicle of the life attribute.*

'*If witnesses derived from DNA, RNA and the amino acids are used, these can immediately give valuable information concerning the three fundamental attributes of the organism: genetic, dynamic and biochemical. Qualitative imbalances in any of these components of the total life of the organism can be detected and evaluated with the help of further witnesses and appropriate measuring scales.*

'*Psionic Medicine stresses the necessity to establish at the outset the basic cause of symptoms before treatment is started. It now becomes clearer that information at genetic level is the first requirement, for it is here that the pattern is established which will influence physical structure, producing abnormalities as a state of disease. This is the level at which consideration must be given to inherited miasms, which derive from the experience of disease in forebears, the commonest of which are the miasms of tuberculosis, syphilis and the sycotic group. This is the point where many of the chronic symptoms of disease in the individual are initiated, irrespective of environment. This is the blueprint stage, the determinant of the form of the organic structure of which protein is ultimately the major con-*

stituent. *The appropriate witness is DNA. With information gained from psionic analysis and with homoeopathic potencies of the correct dynamic order, miasmic disturbances of genetic patterns may be corrected.*

'*It is perhaps necessary to point out here that the symptoms that occur as a result of a particular miasm usually bear no relation to those associated with the original disease in the forebear which gave rise to the miasm genetically. For example, the tubercular miasm can account for the most diverse range of symptoms, including those of asthma, eczema, migraine, diabetes, dental caries, Hodgkin's disease and many other so-called incurable diseases involving various organs and systems.*

'*Protein, and associated substances, taken from the environment in the form of food, provides the material basis — the second attribute. Deficiencies or inferior quality are reflected in the cell substance and may precipitate symptoms. They may also affect vitality. The state of the physical organs and, the conditions of the environment play an important part at this level. The witness used is taken from the amino acids, and their concomitants.*

'*Qualitative changes influencing the building and maintenance processes that constantly go on in the cells are associated with the vital forces. The appropriate witness here is RNA. These changes often occur following acute infections or after the use of their derivatives used in immunisation. They are known in Psionic Medicine as acquired toxins, and again predispose to symptoms apparently unrelated to the infection. They are removed homoeopathically.*

'*Sometimes the acquired toxins may make an impression upon the genetic pattern and establish a chronic predisposition similar to that occurring in inherited miasms. It may be through some such mechanism that the miasmic chain is established. In practice it is found that these acquired toxins may sometimes appear when DNA is used as a witness, especially if all miasms have been previously removed.*'

## Permission

The question of permission is a fundamental ethical principle. Tuning into someone's psi-field should only ever be done with their permission. This actually means permission at different levels.

Firstly, an analysis is only ever done at the request of someone. Usually this is the patient themselves, but sometimes it is a parent, guardian or carer (or owner of a client in veterinary practice). But secondly, after having obtained that verbal or tacit permission, the first question asked in the analysis proper is (something like):

*'May I analyse this patient's specimen?'*

If affirmative, this is followed by (again something like):

*'Can I help this patient?'*

*'Will Psionic Medicine help this patient?'*

*'Am I an appropriate person to treat this patient?'*

*'Should I treat this patient?'*

*'Should I treat this patient now?'*

These questions are extremely important, since they allow the individual's unconscious, their higher self, to express an opinion. It may be that the answer to any of these questions will be no. If this is the case, then the analysis should probably be abandoned, since the permission is being withheld. Experience of practitioners is almost unanimous that, if permission is withheld, then any attempt to treat is likely to be unsuccessful, or even hazardous.

This situation may occur in cases of serious illness, where the individual's higher self may have decided for some reason that this is not what is wanted or needed. Hard though it may be for the individual, relatives or even the practitioner, this wish should be respected.

Sometimes, of course, answers will be affirmative, yet Psionic Medicine is not indicated, in which case further questioning may reveal that the patient at that time will fare better with orthodox medicine, acupuncture or some other therapy.

## Fishing through ice or plumbing the depths

We talked earlier about the process being akin to fishing through ice. This seems a suitable analogy, for the psionic practitioner is not working with direct vision on the individual, but has to use the paranormal dowsing faculty (guided by penetrating and appropriate questioning) to 'feel' his way. He has to differentiate between the different types of 'bites' he perceives, and work out those of greatest significance at that particular moment of time.

Although, as indicated, various techniques are used to show where a problem is, e.g., in the physical, etheric or emotional realms, it is not as simple as that. Just as the fisherman has to develop a feeling for the depth, plumb the depths so to speak, so the practitioner must work out the level at which problems exist, or at which level they are causing major, moderate or minor effects.

Consider a problem in the physical body. The main problem could be a toxin affecting a whole bodily system, or a single organ, or a single tissue, or even a subcellular organelle like a mitochondrion. The problem is that it may only be detectable at certain energetic levels, all others seeming to be normal or unaffected. It is very much a matter of knowing where to look, what to look for and keeping an open mind about finding the unexpected.

## Four stages

The basic framework of the approach, which was originally devised by Laurence, consists of four stages, as follows:

1. The identification of inherited miasms resulting from acute infectious disease in parent or other forebear. This is followed by an assessment of the degree and distribution of the effects of the miasm or miasms throughout the systems, organs and tissues.
2. Identification of the toxic fall-out incurred as a result of acquired infectious illness or other dynamic causes in the individual concerned. A similar determination of degree and distribution is then made. When the diagnosis and analysis have

been completed, an appropriate remedy must be selected psionically, which is indicated as being able to neutralise the toxic emanations identified.

3. The effects on systemic and organ function in relation to protoplasmic changes now affected must be assessed. All other aspects of the new situation both clinically and psionically must be taken into account. Residual gross toxaemia, trace element, mineral or tissue salt[2] deficiency (or failure of utilisation) must be dealt with in the prescription of further remedies, if this is necessary. This is usually accomplished in stages, the most important systems being dealt with first. And not until complete functional balance at all levels is restored can a cure be claimed.

4. Attention may be given at this point to diet and other environmental factors, including psychological deviations that have not responded to the removal of the biological toxins. These may be adversely affecting the patient and offering a threat in the shape of further possible involvement in acute infectious disease.

## Unlocking

Psionic Medicine is essentially an unlocking process whereby one finds the right keys (remedies) to undo the miasms or toxins that are 'locked' into the individual's psi-field. If the wrong keys are selected, then the lock will not open and no result is obtained.

Generally, as one clears a toxin or miasm, the individual experiences improvement in well-being and symptom improvement. Very often, however, there is a transient aggravation of symptoms of the illness or of past problems, which have affected the individual. Again, they do not usually last long.

Here, the use of the onion layer model of miasm and toxin layers is useful in understanding the effect of the remedies.

Each layer represents a toxin or miasm, and is effectively a composite memory of a past illness or trauma, either in the individual or in a parent or forebear. Note that each layer locks in different composite memories. The word 'memory' is important, because in this context there are three types of memory that we need to consider. These are:

*Psychological memory* — This is a memory within the thought field. When it is released the individual recollects something that occurred in the past, possibly associated with the time of origin of that toxin. Often this will manifest as a recollection about a person or place, or as a vivid dream.

*Emotional memory* — This is a memory within the emotional field. When it is released the individual experiences the raw emotion, but often without any associated psychological memory. One just feels irritated, angry, depressed, fearful, jealous, or whatever type of emotion was locked in.

*Body memory* — This is a memory in the etheric body, which is transmitted to the physical body through the etheric–physical interface. It is as if the body itself remembers the physical assault of the trauma or illness, albeit in a modified form. For example, the anatomical site of a past infection, which is recorded in the psi-field as a toxin, will hold a memory. A streptococcal toxin thus often has a body memory in the throat, or there may be a body memory in the bowel of a gastric flu toxin. Or a joint may hold a body memory of a past injury. Effectively, it is as if the physical part actually has a memory of the problem, and is capable of recalling it to produce both symptoms and signs.

When the right key is used to unlock a toxin then the individual may experience emotional, psychological or body memories. Often (but certainly not always) the toxin that is being treated is the most superficial, so that the patient may experience a recurrence of the most recent condition (in a much reduced form), together with other symptoms, depending upon whether emotional or psychological memories are locked in or not.

Figures 22 and 23 may help to explain this. In Figure 22, the homoeopathic remedy is likened to a cricket ball, which we throw into a pond. The surface of the pond is like the energy field. The remedy produces an outward ripple effect, a dispersal effect. Debris is dragged up from the bottom of the pond and dispersed with the ripples. At a certain point, because the remedy is vibrating at the same phase as the layers of toxins (and this is a model of what happens, remember), the ripple will unlock the toxin. This is generally the outermost layer (but certainly not always — each case requiring individual analysis, having unique needs and therefore needing individual treatment).

In Figure 23, as the layer is unlocked, we see how the three types of memory can be released.[3]

Indeed, this model often explains the mechanism of Hering's Law,[4] the direction of cure, which is one of the oft-quoted (*yet inconsistent*) phenomena of homoeopathy.[5]

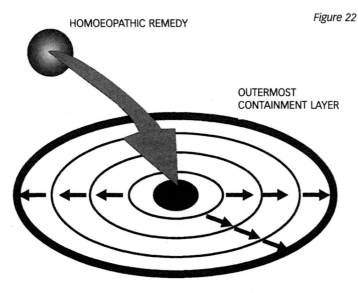

HOMOEOPATHIC REMEDY

*Figure 22*

OUTERMOST
CONTAINMENT LAYER

HOMOEOPATHIC ACTIVATION CAUSING
OUTWARD DISPERAL AND UNLOCKING EFFECT

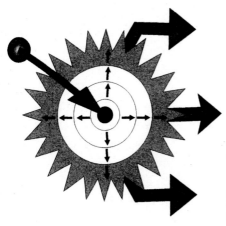

EMOTIONAL MEMORY
e.g. jealousy, anger, depression, anxiety

— without any obvious trigger, but relates to a past emotion

PSYCHOLOGICAL MEMORY
e.g. flashbacks, sudden recollections, or vivid dreams of people, events and past experiences or traumas

BODY MEMORY
e.g. pain, breathlessness, alteration in function, skin rash

— without any obvious trigger, but relates to a past physical symptom or condition

HOMOEOPATHIC ACTIVATION CAUSING
OUTWARD DISPERAL AND UNLOCKING EFFECT                    *Figure 23*

At other times, the removal of one layer allows the next layer to begin to agitate, which means that emotional, psychological and physical memories from that layer may flare up transiently.

It can be seen, therefore, that the layers are not unlike a nest of locked Russian dolls. As each one is opened it allows memories (of the three types — all, only two or possibly only one) to flare up transiently. The next one may bring entirely different symptoms, so the progress may be quite an adventure in healing for the individual. But a healing process it is likely to be, since the individual's natural healing abilities are being hampered by these layers. Remove them and the natural healing process begins.

The number of treatments that each person needs is variable. Some people may need a single treatment while others seem to have a succession of layers that need to be gently worked through. In the next chapter, in order to give the reader a flavour of the diversity of problems that psionic medicine can deal with, we will look at a few cases that have been recorded over the years in the *Journal of the Psionic Medical Society and the Institute of Psionic Medicine.*

## A summary from Carl Upton

To understand the Psionic Medicine approach it is necessary to extend one's thinking beyond the ideas of conventional acceptance; but this does not mean that Psionic Medicine is a mere theory. On the contrary, it is of the greatest practical value, once its techniques have been mastered, as is proved by its record of successes, some of which are detailed in the next chapter.

As has been repeatedly emphasised, the analysis and treatment is essentially individual, not relying on standardised diagnosis and treatment; nor does it involve animal experimentation. There is today much interest in transplant and 'spare part' surgery. But such techniques, with their moral issues and considerable expenditure of manpower and resources, might well be avoided by psionic analysis earlier in life, before irreversible damage has occurred.

Similarly, mental illness could be reduced extensively. It was Laurence's experience that a large percentage of cases in this category are due to inherited miasms and acquired toxins — possibly aggravated by external conditions, including modern drugs, but not necessarily primarily caused by them.

Moreover, psionic techniques can be used to test the effect of conventional drugs on the individual vitality. They also provide a means of checking intolerance and sensitivity to aluminium, fluoride, mercury, radiation and other toxic factors with which the individual may come into contact; and if these are present, they may be neutralised.

If some of the resources at present squandered on the attempted amelioration of physical symptoms could be diverted to the study of the dynamic causes of illness, new horizons would appear in medical research which could lead to a more comprehensive health service.

[1] Psionic witnesses usually consist of 1g vials containing tablets or granules treated with a particular homoeopathic potency of the desired sample.

[2] The Biochemic Tissue Salts are a group of inorganic compounds which are all present in the human body, and which have particular vital metabolic functions. A whole system of therapeutics, coined 'Biochemics' was devised by Dr William H. Schuessler who started publishing his work in 1837. There are 12 basic biochemic tissue salts and 18 special combinations (available over the counter and used around the world) which are available for self-help. They are sometimes referred to as the Schuessler Salts.

[3] Sometimes patients also feel an additional awareness, as if they become more intuitive for a short period of time. This would seem to come about because the containment layer is breached, allowing greater access to the psi-field.

[4] Hering's Law, formulated by Constantine Hering, see Chapter 5. Essentially, it states that a cure is effected: from above downwards, from within outwards, from major to lesser organs, and it takes place in reverse order of appearance of symptoms.

[5] A reason why the Law is not constant is because the remedy is probably working from within outwards, like the wave in Figure 22. The remedy chosen will possibly also have a spectrum of activity broader than that of the single toxin. This being the case it will often have a positive effect on other layers as it works its way to the layer most in need of removal. Thus, memories of the three types may be stimulated from the other layers in addition to the one it is unlocking.

# 12

# Psionic Medicine in Practice

'The physician's high and only mission is to restore the sick to health, to cure as it is termed.'

**First aphorism, Organon of Medicine**
**Samuel Hahnemann**

'Physicians, when the cause of disease is discovered, consider that the cure is discovered.'

**Cicero**

'The physician treats, nature makes well.'

**Quintilian**

Psionic Medicine is not a panacea.[1] Its aim is to seek the cause of the illness and remove it. The individual's self-regulatory functions, the healing power of nature in other words, are always striving to make the best efforts that they can, but miasms, toxins and other traumas can interfere with this in a manner of ways, as we have seen in the last chapter. Psionic Medicine is an integrative method, which links both orthodox medicine and homoeopathy. Sometimes it will be the only method that is necessary and sometimes it will work in conjunction with other methods. At the very least, it will clear the toxic load that acts as a brake on the natural self-healing and self-regulating functions of the individual, so that the individual will respond better to other methods.

As an example of this, it is not unusual to see someone who has failed to respond to some method of treatment, only for them to have a course of psionic treatment, which then allows the original treatment to work. One often sees this in chronic back complaints that do not respond to physiotherapy, acupuncture or chiropractic until they have had a toxic load removed.

## Psionic practice profile

People from all walks of life find their way to Psionic Medicine. The nature of the discipline and the method of analysis is such that many practitioners have patients coming to them from all over the world. Some are self-referred, while others are referred by other health practitioners in order to achieve clearance of toxic loads, such as mentioned above.

Although every psionic practitioner tends to be a generalist, each will have specific areas of interest and expertise. Also, while all will have been trained in the Laurence-Upton technique, it is likely that each will have brought their own insights to the approach so that they are liable to have an individual way of practising. For all these reasons the profile of patients treated is likely to be different from practitioner to practitioner. Having said that, it is worth looking at the broad profile of cases that presented in one practice over a year.

Firstly, the presenting complaint (Figure 24). We see here that cancers, chronic fatigue, respiratory, rheumatological and gastro-intestinal diseases account for about 60 per cent of the caseload. The relatively low figure of six per cent for psychological complaints is possibly less than one would imagine, but it has to be noted that these are figures for the presenting complaint. Practice actually demonstrates that emotional and psychological components are common. Indeed, one would say that most people who are suffering from ill health will at the very least feel anxious.

An age-sex breakdown (Figure 25) shows that more females than males consult but, again, this is true across the board: the figures are similar in orthodox general practice. Respiratory

PRESENTING COMPLAINT

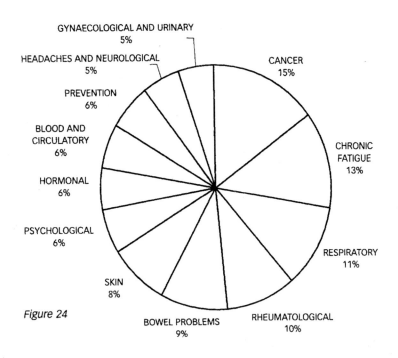

Figure 24

Figure 25          SEX DIFFERENCES BETWEEN MAIN GROUPS

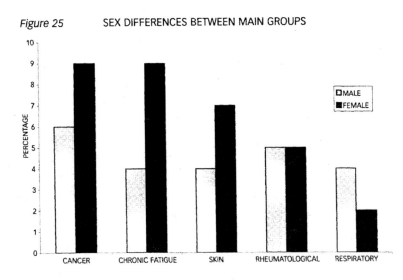

complaints are more common in males, whereas more females consult about chronic fatigue and skin problems.

When we look at the miasms and toxins found at *first* analysis (Figure 26), the significance of the tubercular miasms, and the acquired toxin of measles is immediately apparent. Metal toxicity is predominantly caused by aluminium, with mercury coming second.

MIASMS AND TOXINS FOUND AT FIRST ANALYSIS

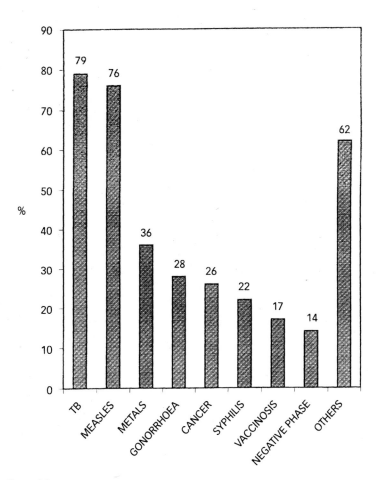

Figure 26

An analysis of the 'other' group, which occurs in 60 per cent of cases, is worth a closer look (Figure 27). This is predominantly made up of bacterial- and viral-acquired toxins, but here we also find mineral and electrolyte anomalies, sensitivity to geopathic stress (which includes underground streams, electric fields, and mobile phone problems), allergies and other problems.

The question of allergies is interesting, because the allergy, per se, is often not the cause of the problem, but is rather more usually a manifestation of the body's struggle with its toxic load. This often surprises people who have been informed that their allergic tendency (usually to foods) is the source of their problem.

At this point it is worth considering how some of these miasms and toxins can affect the individual. Again, partly to document

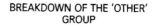

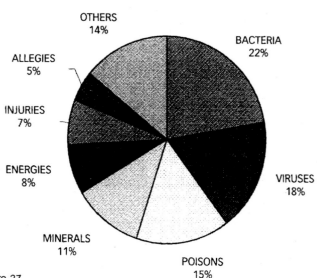

BREAKDOWN OF THE 'OTHER'
GROUP

OTHERS
14%

BACTERIA
22%

ALLEGIES
5%

INJURIES
7%

ENERGIES
8%

VIRUSES
18%

MINERALS
11%

POISONS
15%

*Figure 27*

this as an original piece of work, here follows a paper by Carl Upton, originally published as an appendix to the second edition of this book.

NB: For bioplasm, read personal psi-field.

## Commentary by Carl Upton on the bioplasm and associated clinical indications

Medical science deals very competently with structural defects and it is customarily assumed that physiological disorders can be remedied by similar mechanistic methods. All too often, however, such treatment is only partially successful. A state of malaise may persist, not necessarily in the same form, while if the illness has become chronic it may fail altogether to respond to orthodox treatment. It becomes clear that subtle changes and processes may be taking place, which are not perceived by conventional means.

It is with these deeper causes that Psionic Medicine is concerned. They arise from disturbances in the unseen pattern of influences which determines all physical manifestations. These distortions create a variety of chemical and physical effects and may eventually produce physical symptoms. The existence of this underlying pattern is now accepted in the scientific world in which it has become known as the 'bioplasm'.

By its very nature the bioplasm cannot be directly observed, nor can its properties be assessed by the yardsticks of material perception and knowledge, but its presence and potentialities can be discerned by the deeper levels of the mind employing faculties beyond the range of the ordinary physical senses. This creates a new dimension of understanding, which can then be developed by practical experience.

First of all, we have to consider the relationship that exists between the bioplasm and physical matter. It is clear that it is a relationship between dynamic potentiality and functional process. The bioplasm would appear to possess properties of attraction, repulsion and memory which can create 'crystallisations' of specific form and purpose from the raw materials that surround it in the physical world. Thus the bioplasm relative to a particular human being builds and maintains the organic structure, and influences the physiological behaviour of that individual. Only essential changes in the bioplasm can produce definitive modifications in the external organic manifestation.

It seems, moreover, that different scales of time, as well as space, are involved, analogous perhaps to the different orbits in the galaxies and their relative influences. One cycle in the overall pattern may involve a multiplicity of subsidiary cycles. The reproduction of similar cells which occurs throughout the life of the individual represents a process of recurrence at the physical level reflecting a single imprint of the bioplasmic pattern. This implies that any aberration in the bioplasm may produce a recurrent and sustained deviation in cell behaviour, which may be the cause of chronic symptoms of ill health.

Furthermore, the human being does not live in a state of isolation – globally or organically. Reciprocal influences are constantly at play, and these may have both essential and superficial results. At the superficial level it is relatively easy to determine a cause and effect relationship, both temporally and spatially. The spread of an acute infection or the disability arising from an injury are plain to see, but when the subtler and normally unseen processes are concerned the connections are not so readily discerned: they reside in the bioplasm.

One bioplasmic state can affect another. For instance, the bioplasm of a human being may be influenced by that of a microorganism, but because of the differing time and space scales the result is quite different from the material association such as occurs in an acute infection. Indeed, at the bioplasmic level changes may occur of an essential nature, which bring results that do not coincide with familiar physical parameters. In certain cases, the subtle bioplasmic influence may carry over several generations, constituting what the homoeopath calls a 'miasm'.

Considerable variations occur in symptom patterns due to the effects of changes in the bioplasm. Some bioplasmic states are long-lived. Others are relatively transient and 'decay' in a matter of weeks or months. A reversion to normal may then take place, but an apparent resolution of external symptoms does not necessarily mean that the vital dynamis has again reverted to balance. Indeed, in the course of time a totally new set of symptoms may appear and for no obvious reason. Only an examination of the bioplasm can reveal the cause.

In addition to influences from lower forms of life, which cause changes in the bioplasm and consequent clinical effects, there are also influences from less material realms. For example, the bioplasm may be influenced by the psychic processes, which can just as readily produce changes which ultimately become manifest at the physical level; and it is known that negative psychological states render the body more vulnerable to infection.

Conversely, good psychological states confer a certain degree of immunity and the possibilities, in general, must not be seen only in their negative aspects. The very principles, laws and processes involved bear also the potentiality of healing. Nature in her bounty makes available an extensive range of influences that may bring about a state of reconciliation and consequent health, if they are properly understood. Considerable use of these natural facilities is made in homeopathic and psionic medical practice.

It is evident that exploration of the bioplasmic realm requires a patient and individual approach, which cannot be reduced to a routine basis. Nevertheless, from observations over an extended period it has been possible to formulate certain approximate correlations between bioplasmic states and associated clinical symptoms. These can be no more than a guide to the areas of derangement, which must then be examined by psionic investigation.

A further difficulty is that since there are no specific terms available to indicate states of the vital dynamis or bioplasm the only option is to use the terms which define the clinical manifestation. Thus, when the tubercular state is mentioned it does not refer to an acute infection or bacillus, but to the observed condition of the bioplasm in the particular circumstances; and, be it noted, it may be associated with a set of symptoms which in the ordinary way could appear quite irrelevant. Similarly, the word toxin in this context refers to a bioplasmic disturbance and not to a clinical manifestation.

With this understanding, Table 1, setting out some correlations observed over many years, may provide a practical guide to possible areas of search.

The classical 'miasms' have general indications as follows:

Psora: Skin itch. Functional disturbance of organs and unusual objective sensations.

Sycosis: Overgrowth of tissue, warts, moles and papillomata, gouty concretions and osteoarthritis, pelvic inflammations and discharges.

Syphilis: All distortions of body structure and function. Destruction of tissues. Varicose veins, hernias and dental malocclusion. Psychogenic imbalance.

## Negative phase

A disorder, which arises from an attenuation of the bioplasm, is known as 'negative phase'. It differs from the state of condensation that occurs when toxins and miasms are present. It relates to over-activity of the property of repulsion in the bioplasm. Clinical indications are vital depletion associated with over-expansion of protein. Hypoglycaemia. Lethargy. Loss of physical and psychological coordination. Wandering and indeterminate pains. Tends to follow injury or psychological trauma and major surgery. It may be transient but where the degree of disturbance is intense or prolonged it can persist over long periods and the cause goes unrecognised. When it is present the likelihood of infection is often increased.

## NOTE ON NEGATIVE PHASE

The above description of negative phase was, as mentioned earlier, Carl Upton's concept. Current psionic practioners would concede that it describes it in part, but would say that it is an entirely more complicated state of affairs than Carl envisaged.

Dr George Laurence often found a relative deficiency in body phosphorus, which may account for the general weariness which so often accompanies negative phase. This has often been confirmed by current practitioners.

Dr Gordon Flint, the President of the Institute, also feels that, because negative phase masks any other toxic factor which may be present and blocks most forms of treatment, it is always important to test again, when specific therapy has been selected, in order to identify any such masked toxin and deal with it in its own right.

In the clinical setting, when describing it to a patient, Dr Flint compares it with the person, in imagination, standing very close to the edge of a cliff. In normal circumstances, with a good head for heights, this will not cause any distress. In the negative state, however, the cloud around them is so thick that they cannot see their hand in front of their face and they have no idea where the cliff edge is, other than that it is very close. They cannot see through the cloud to seek help and potential help cannot see through the cloud to offer it. The only options are: 1) To remain very still until the cloud lifts, which it will, even if it takes days or weeks, or 2) Specific treatment can be selected which will clear the cloud much more quickly, so that the cliff edge being obvious, a safe pathway can be chosen away from it, avoiding any boulders, etc., which might represent other toxic factors, previously masked by the cloud.

Regarding the finding of hypoglycaemia which Carl Upton quotes, Dr Flint believes that this is not a constant or a diagnostic finding in itself. Using his background in chemistry, he has conducted much research into acid-base balance, which may have a bearing upon relative blood sugar levels.

Table 1 was compiled by Carl Upton and must not be regarded as a definitive or complete listing of miasms and toxins, or their effects. There are many more to be found, but these are all still very common and more or less represent a basic listing. Please also see the tables in Chapter Six, by Dr Farley Spink, and in Chapter Fourteen, by Mr Mark Elliott.

### Tubercular miasm or toxin
Possible clinical manifestations are many and diverse. They include asthma, eczema, migraine, diabetes, Hodgkin's disease. Also temperamental instability, especially in childhood, dental caries, glandular disturbance and various functional disabilities. A mild and artistic nature prevails.

### Syphilis miasm or toxin
This is related to a number of neurological and psychotic conditions affecting nervous function and psychological behaviour. Miscarriage, spontaneous abortion, premature birth, failure to conceive and many physical and behavioural deformities including Down's syndrome, multiple sclerosis, the ataxias and loss of function. Violent, aggressive temperament with a tendency to dominate and tyrannise.

### Gonorrhoea toxin
Overgrowth of tissue, warts, moles, papillomata, tumour formation are often related to this state. Osteoarthritis, gout and catarrhal genito-urinary discharges; prostatic conditions are often associated. By nature tendency to be withdrawn and self centred.

### Measles toxin
Skin complaints and disturbances of cardio-vascular, mucosal and hard tissues. When associated with the tubercular state, which it often is, this toxin may emphasise the clinical effects and unless cleared tends to lock in and make its removal more difficult.

### Staphylococcus aureus
The residual toxins may lead to chronic respiratory or gastro-enteric symptoms. Sinusitis, tonsillitis, bronchitis that do not respond to conventional treatment, usually antibiotic, frequently indicate the presence of this toxin. Chronic gall-bladder inflammation and other disturbances of the portal system may also be associated.

### Staphylococcus albus
Skin complaints, boils, carbuncles suggest this toxin.

### Streptococcus
Cardiovascular, musculoskeletal and neurological conditions may be related. Meninges and mucous membranes may also be involved. Throat infections.

### Influenza
Depression, sometimes persisting over long periods. Respiratory and gastroenteric disturbances. Negative emotional states, lassitude and lack of energy can also be related.

### Micrococcus catarrhalis
Chronic sinusitis, rhinitis.

### E. coli
Chronic and recurrent inflammation of genito-urinary tract. Cystitis, kidney complaints, prostatitis. Also bowel problems and tooth disorders.

### Atypical coli bacilli
Can affect all systems with evidence of an attempt on the part of the organism to discharge toxic substances. Portal, genito-urinary, respiratory, musculoskeletal, lymphatic and cutaneous channels may be involved. Physical and mental strain may be associated.

### Glandular fever
Lymphatic abnormalities and recurrent debilitation.

### Malaria
Blood disorders, debility, depression and psychological disturbances.

### Amoebic dysentery
Liver complaints and chronic digestive problems often persisting over long periods. General debility.

### Poliomyelitis
Intractable constipation. Disordered muscular function leading to deformity. Local instability.

### Aluminium
Skin, digestive and neurological complaints. Varicose ulcers. Peptic ulceration, hiatus hernia and oesophagitis. Inflammatory bowel disease.

### Vaccination
Fibrous growths, tumours, warts. Skin, breast and genito-urinary system are common sites of abnormalities.

### Paratyphoid
Musculoskeletal and digestive disorders.

### Whooping cough
Chronic chest complaints.

### Salmonella
Chronic digestive complaints. Debility.

### Herpes Zoster
Persistent skin lesion and pain. Debility.

### Brucellosis
Chronic ill health affecting many systems and leaving the patient slow to recover.

### Internal parasites
General toxaemia which may affect any organ and create general irritation and debility. Portal and genito-urinary systems principally affected.

### Tropical parasites
Persistent digestive disorders and disturbances of fibrous tissues through chronic toxaemia.

On a pH scale, he finds that the average female, of whatever age, appears to function best against a background pH (derived by radiesthetic testing) of 7.1, while males are more on the alkaline side at pH 7.5. The true ME sufferers seem to be functioning against an acidic background pH of 6.5 (when they may experience relative hypoglycaemia). On the other hand, those people in negative phase may be operating, inefficiently, at an alkaline pH of 8.0.

(Please also see the section on *Positive or negative response* in Chapter Six, on Miasms and Toxins, by Dr Farley Spink.)

## Clinical cases

It is now worth spending some time looking at what sort of conditions are seen in psionic practice, and get some flavour of the sort of treatments given.

The following cases have been selected from previously published papers in the *Journal of the Psionic Medical Society*. They are not arranged in chronological order, but loosely by presenting complaint. This is quite deliberate, since cases treated by Dr George Laurence and Mr Carl Upton appear alongside those of current practitioners.

### MIGRAINE

This condition is extremely common nowadays. Conventional treatment consists of using medication to deal with severe, occasional attacks, or using prophylactic treatment if the attacks are very frequent. Sufferers will know how debilitating it can be.

Psionic analysis has established that the effects are the result of miasmatic disturbances, either hereditary or acquired, and that by appropriate treatment the malady can often be permanently cured.

Relatively mild cases are usually found to arise from unsuspected acquired toxins. One example is a lady who had suffered from recurring headaches, which at the age of 43 were becoming intolerable. Psionic analysis disclosed a *malaria toxin*, a hangover from an attack in her childhood. Removal of this toxin effected a complete cure.

### Mr C.W., aged 57

The onset of migraine with severe headaches, nausea and vomiting, occurred at approximately 18 years of age.

Attacks, which were often associated with events in which an element of emotional strain was involved, usually lasted for some hours and responded to light sedation and sleep. With advancing years the duration of the attacks increased until the usual pattern was extended over three days, often commencing on awakening in the morning.

For some years the attacks appeared to be linked in some sort of rhythmic pattern, often occurring at weekends. Certain foods were thought to increase susceptibility. The disrupting effect of the disease drove the patient to seek all forms of treatment in an attempt to find relief. Orthodox medication with ergotamine tartrate and other drugs failed to bring results, and resort had to be made to strong sedatives containing codeine, plus attempts to remain quiet in a darkened room.

In 1966 a psionic medical diagnosis was undertaken which disclosed the existence of *tubercular miasms* of both strains — *Bovine* and *Koch*. Treatment was commenced and continued over a period of several weeks. Since that time there has been no recurrence of the characteristic attacks. Occasional headaches, following periods of stress, have occurred but have responded immediately to mild sedation.

### Mr S.C.W.S., aged 44

The patient reported that he had had frequent attacks of migraine over 25 years, latterly several times a week. He also complained of continual tiredness. The first signs of an attack were flashing lights on one side, followed by pain down the side of the head, a feeling of sickness and then vomiting on most occasions. Whilst an attack was in progress there was a dislike of bright light. The duration of the attack was usually about five hours.

A psionic diagnosis revealed the *double tubercular miasm* and a *meningeal imbalance*. There was also a *measles toxin*. Treatment was started with a view to eliminating inherited and acquired toxic factors and an immediate reduction in frequency and intensity of attack occurred. Five months later the patient wrote to say, 'I have now finished my last course of tablets. Since my last report to you I am pleased to tell you that I have had no attacks of migraine at all.'

### Mrs X., aged 45

This patient had severe migraines since she started to menstruate at 13, together with various allergies, for which she had tried every form of treatment with no lasting relief.

She proved to be a very difficult case to treat, as the basic cause was found to be *three hereditary miasms (including the double tubercular miasms)*, which were very difficult to dislodge; in fact it was not until she had five courses of basic treatment that the miasms were finally eliminated.

There were homoeopathic aggravations, but on the whole the symptoms slowly became less severe, until four months after commencing treatment she could report she hoped she had turned a corner.

Treatment was continued on and off for another six months, by which time she was very much better in every way. She has had treatment for other minor ailments, which have cropped up as a result of foreign travel, but the original migraines and allergic symptoms are now a thing of the past.

### Mr J.W., aged 20

This case is typical of many migraine sufferers, both symptomatically and causatively. The patient complained of frequent and severe attacks of headache and photophobia, usually at weekly intervals. The attack lasted for one or two days and was accompanied by the characteristic nausea. There were no other outstanding symptoms apart from a high incidence of dental caries.

Psionic analysis revealed *both tubercular miasms* and activity of *Sycotic co.*, a non-lactose fermenting bowel organism usually associated with the catarrhal state.

Treatment was initiated to remove the miasms and the toxin, and the response was rapid, the symptoms subsiding within a few weeks. A little later the patient contracted influenza, which was given appropriate homoeopathic treatment and which led to a short period in the *negative phase*, with characteristic feeling of tiredness and depression. Some three months after the first treatment for the removal of the miasms some bronchial symptoms appeared, and these were found to be associated with *Staphylo-coccus aureus* infection. When this was cleared the patient required no further treatment and has remained well and symptom-free since.

## RAYNAUD'S SYNDROME

This is a vasospastic condition mainly affecting the hands, but sometimes the feet as well. Attacks are often precipitated by cold and sometimes by motion (especially vibration) but sometimes they are quite random. Attacks are characterised by episodes of arteriolar spasm, which produces white, cold and painful fingers and hands. Over minutes to hours the fingers can go cyanotic (blue or purple, through diminished oxygen being supplied to the tissues). Ultimately, it ends with a red flushing phase.

When the condition is not associated with any underlying disorder, it is termed Raynaud's syndrome, and skin changes are not seen. This is commonest in young women.

When the condition is associated with an underlying condition it is termed Raynaud's phenomenon. This can occur in people with collagen diseases, protein abnormalities, or in occupational vibrational trauma.

Psionic treatment can often produce amazing results.

### Ms R.W., aged 32

This lady of Afro-Caribbean ancestry had suffered from cold hands all of her life. This had prevented her playing sport at school, or spending any time more than was necessary out of doors during the winter. Only in the summer months was she able to discard her gloves. Even then, swimming was an activity she avoided, since even the temperature of an ordinary swimming pool could trigger an attack.

At the age of 30 years she had a psionic analysis, which revealed an inherited *leprosy toxin*. After treatment with the nosode and some further supporting homoeopathic remedies the problem receded considerably.

That winter she was overjoyed to go snowballing with a nephew, without gloves.

### Mr A.S., aged 54

This man had been forced to give up his work in a heavy industry, owing to the development of 'white finger', an occupational Raynaud's phenomenon. A heavy smoker, he had been advised to stop, and successfully did so, but without relief of the problem.

A psionic analysis showed the presence of an acquired *proteus toxin*. Once this was cleared, together with a *double inherited tubercular miasm*, his symptoms improved. Again with further supportive homoeopathic treatment his condition all but disappeared.

## ASTHMA AND RELATED CONDITIONS

Asthma and eczema are increasingly common conditions. They are often deep-seated, requiring prolonged homoeopathic medication, but psionic treatment is often ultimately successful.

### M.H., aged 9

This was a young boy who had been troubled with asthma and recurring eczema since the age of six months. It was not until he was nine years old that his parents sought the advice of a psionic practitioner, who discovered two underlying miasms — *TK* (tubercular Koch miasm) and *poliomyelitis*. After two and a half months the poliomyelitis miasm was eliminated, and the TK miasm greatly reduced, but a *TB* (tubercular bovine miasm) was then uncovered, together with one of *pertussis* (whooping cough).

The indicated treatment was given for a further six months, but although the pertussis miasm disappeared at once, and the readings for TK and TB were reduced, the miasms remained remarkably resistant; and it was not until another six months later that they were cleared. By then he developed a *staphylococcus aureus* infection and, surprisingly, the miasms became active for a further two months before disappearing completely.

One year at school, during the earlier part of which he was having continuous treatment, his health improved considerably and he had no time off, but on returning home for the summer holidays his wheeziness returned. This was assumed to be due to emotional excitement, but after further homoeopathic treatment it subsided, and on his Christmas holiday there was no recurrence, despite an influenza epidemic at the time.

The following year his father wrote, 'It is very apparent that the treatment given my son has been progressively successful in its results. His health is now excellent and he has not lost any time from school, whilst he is acquitting himself well academically and more than holding his own with the other boys.'

This case brings out an important fact, namely that in these deep-seated chronic conditions, even though the underlying causal factors are eliminated, a residual pattern appears to remain temporarily, and this can be activated by extraneous toxic and emotional factors, as in this case, where emotion could bring on the attacks of wheeziness.

### N.T., aged 7

This child had had asthma practically all his life; and he continually missed school and was a great worry to his mother who could do little for his obvious distress.

Psionic analysis showed the usual *TB/TK miasms* together with a *measles toxin*. After two courses of treatment his mother reported that he had had no colds and no return of his asthma, whereas previously a cold always produced a severe attack. He has not looked back, and his mother says that the cure has changed both their lives.

### Mrs F.M.H., aged 60

This patient had suffered attacks of asthma since she was about 44 years old, with increasing intensity. She had been a delicate child, with a tendency to chest trouble. She complained of constant breathlessness and recurrent bronchitis. Constipation and increase of girth at diaphragm level were also featured. There was incipient cataract. Operations for the removal of gall bladder and appendix had been performed.

A psionic medical diagnosis was carried out in 1968 and this indicated the presence of the *double tubercular miasm* with the acquired toxins resulting from *streptococcus* infection and *malaria*. A later analysis showed the patient to be sensitive to *aluminium* used in cooking.

Several courses of homoeopathic medicines were necessary, the final course being in April 1969, when an *atypical bacillus coli bowel organism* was present. After this was cleared the patient reported a good state of general health and complete freedom from asthma and chest trouble. The improvement has been maintained.

This case illustrates the diversity of symptoms that can occur through the presence of mixed miasms and acquired toxins. It also shows how in some cases the final response of the organism in cure produces changes in the bowel flora; and once this is corrected the case proceeds to a satisfactory conclusion.

### Mrs I.C., aged 49

This was a case of chronic dermatitis of arms and legs, which failed to respond to orthodox medical treatment. Various forms of skin lesions were present, which had been treated by both her general medical practitioner and the local consultant dermatologist over three years without effect. As the patient was engaged in domestic work using detergents it was thought that this might have some bearing and protective gloves had been advised, but again with no effect. The trouble appeared to be spreading and the patient was becoming desperate.

On the advice of her employer she agreed to psionic medical analysis. This showed that inherited miasms of *syphilis* and *tuberculosis* were present, as well as toxins of *staphylococcus* and *aluminium*. The indicated homoeopathic medicines were prescribed and there was immediate improvement. After three courses of medicine all lesions had completely cleared and the skin was perfectly normal. The patient had continued her domestic work throughout. Two years on, the skin was still normal.

### M.S.R., aged 7

This child had measles at 20 months and bronchitis when she was two years old, followed shortly afterwards by a further attack, and a month later, pneumonia.

Thereafter she had recurring attacks of asthma. Every cold always seemed to develop into this, and was only relieved by a coal tar vaporizer and a bronchodilator syrup. Each attack would last for about a week, and she was frequently rushed into hospital.

When she was nearly seven, further advice was sought. A psionic analysis showed that the underlying factors of her illness were *TB/TK miasms* and the acquired *measles* toxin. The indicated treatment was given, which at first increased the asthma (homoeopathic aggravation), but she quickly recovered. With further treatment the miasms and toxin factors disappeared, and by the following spring, in spite of a bad cold in the late winter, she became free of her asthma and was in good health and has remained so.

#### ALLERGIES AND ALUMINIUM SENSITIVITY

Affections of the skin are of frequent occurrence and are often difficult to diagnose. They may be due to allergic conditions but in many instances are the result of toxins acquired from the inimical energies in aluminium.

Aluminium also seems to have a deleterious effect upon the cardio-vascular, gastrointestinal and nervous systems.

Aluminium is used widely in cooking utensils, in foods, in beauty preparations, deodorants and in canning.

### Mrs D.M., aged 40

The complaint in this case was of recurring patches of dry skin, especially on the face, which sometimes became red and irritable.

The onset was usually quite unexpected and rapid. There was also at the same time a persistent breakdown of the skin at the margin of the nostrils on one side with a persistent ulceration. The eye was also sometimes affected. There were no miasms or toxins associated with infectious illness, since these had been removed previously. A further, rather wider analysis showed that the patient was sensitive to cat hair. Accordingly, during an attack, potentised cat hair was prescribed as the remedy and at the second dose the skin was cleared completely.

After several weeks, however, there was a further eruption with similar skin characteristics. On this occasion a further dose of cat hair failed to be effective. A yet more comprehensive analysis showed a sensitivity to *primula* and indeed it was confirmed that a primula was present in the house. Attention having been drawn to this new possibility, careful observation showed that in fact when she touched the primula, she had an immediate skin reaction. Homoeopathic primula was prescribed and the plant removed. There have been no further complaints.

This case illustrates the fact that when the basic constitutional predispositions are eliminated it does not necessarily follow that residual effects are clear. They may persist and require attention for some time.

### Mrs W.T., aged 40

This patient had suffered from a chronic area of ulceration on her right leg for three years. This did not respond to any form of orthodox medication. She had a yellowish complexion and said that she had had a history of pyelitis for ten years. She also complained of an eye lesion, which was said to be of tropical origin.

Psionic analysis revealed the presence of the *double tubercular miasm*, together with acquired *E. coli toxin*, and *aluminium poisoning*. Appropriate treatment was commenced and the patient was advised to discard all aluminium utensils. There was a good response to the initial medication, which was continued at intervals with further improvement. After four months the patient reported complete recovery with no vestige of the former skin condition.

### Miss J., aged 27

This lady had had ulcerative colitis for three years when she was first seen. Conventional medication had made her feel generally unwell. She was fed up with the daily rectal steroids, though they did seem to control her symptoms. She was particularly concerned about the frequent hospital check-ups and invasive investigations.

On psionic analysis she was found to have an *aluminium toxin* as well as *both tubercular toxins* and a *candida albicans toxin*. After these were cleared she needed considerable rebalancing of the portal system and clearance of a *chlamydia toxin*. It was not until a second aluminium clearance that she became totally free from symptoms. She remains so, although she must avoid aluminium as far as possible. Recognising and dealing with the underlying causes of her illness has resulted in great improvement in her general physical and psychological well-being.

### Mr I.B.M.C., aged 56

In this case there had been a colon imbalance for 12 years. It was originally associated with a pain in the groin and testicles. He had some symptoms of migraine. His appetite was small. He had a history of diphtheria as a child.

Psionic analysis showed the *double tubercular miasms*, together with the *acquired measles toxin* and an *aluminium toxin*. Three prescriptions were given over a four-month period with good result. The patient, who had been using aluminium extensively, changed all utensils in the kitchen to enamel and stainless steel, and avoided aluminium as much as possible.

Later that year the patient noted a slight recurrence, which analysis showed to be due to the aluminium toxin. This was then cleared again.

Some time later, the patient wrote to say he had worked out that the source of aluminium exposure had been frozen foods. These had been previously prepared in an aluminium pressure cooker.

## PSYCHOLOGICAL CONDITIONS

There is often great scope for psionic analysis in this field. Psionic treatment has had considerable success in the treatment of anxiety, depression, phobic states and even psychotic conditions, such as schizophrenia and manic-depressive illness.

### Mrs E.P., aged 44

This patient had a record of outbursts of vituperation and violence. In 1966, when she was 41, she started a transport business which grew so rapidly that she became heavily overburdened with problems, and in 1968 she had a 'breakdown', becoming withdrawn, intent on psychic matters and spiritualism, with various psychotic manifestations and symptoms, which were eventually diagnosed as schizophrenia. But by this time she had so lost touch with reality that she had landed herself and her husband in crippling debt. Her condition deteriorated and by 1970 she took to her bed with fantasies and delusions of her identity. She was finally taken to a mental hospital but refused treatment and left after two days.

Her husband, in desperation, asked for homoeopathic treatment on psionic medical indications. The analysis showed both *syphilitic* and *tubercular miasms* particularly affecting her brain and central nervous system, but in addition she had an *atypical bacillus coli* in the bowel (probably the result of previous use of antibiotics), and cellular dehydration.

The treatment indicated and prescribed was in four stages, but administration proved very difficult and at times appeared hopeless, as the patient chain-smoked, drank tea and coffee as well as wine at the time of taking the remedies, regardless of advice to the contrary, and later refused all treatment at two periods midway between the second and third stages.

In April her condition deteriorated to the point that she required hospital admission and treatment. However, on returning home, she stopped all treatment and again deteriorated, eventually taking to her bed. Fortunately, at this point she agreed to take her homoeopathic treatment, and the third stage was completed. She still continued to drink, since she was unable to sleep.

The fourth stage of treatment was then begun. After the first powder she went to bed and slept soundly. In succeeding days she drank less, and continued to sleep well. On the sixth powder (on the fourteenth day) she stated that she felt well, and that she thought she had passed a crisis.

She continued to improve all round and by the end of August she went with her small son and her mother to the south coast. When her husband joined her for the weekend, he found her 'healthy, cheerful and normal'. A psionic analysis a month later found that at last she was clear of all miasms and toxic factors.

From this point she gradually moved stage by stage back to normal life. Her humour and quick intelligence returned. She became increasingly physically active and her husband stated that 'the change is so striking as to make the past year or two seem unreal.'

Two years on, she had returned to business, and has taken up all her old hobbies. Effectively, she had left her illness and all it stood for behind her.

### Miss R.F., aged 35

This case presented with phobic fear of vomiting. This is a social phobia, which usually responds well to hypnotherapy. However, the patient, although a good hypnotic subject, was still subject to the phobic fear in certain conditions. She agreed to have a psionic analysis performed, which showed *Dys Co* to be present.

Two treatments dealt with the problem.

There are countless other cases recorded in the literature of the Psionic Medical Society, but this selection was chosen to show the range of conditions which are amenable to the psionic approach.

[1] Panacea, a universal remedy or cure-all, from the Greek 'panakeia' — 'pan' meaning 'all' and 'akeisthai' 'to heal', from 'akos' meaning 'remedy'.

In Greek mythology Asclepius, the god of healing had several daughters, his favourites being Hygieia and Panacea. The original Hippocratic oath begins 'I swear by Apollo, by Hygieia, by Panacea and all the gods and goddesses of the pantheon...'

# 13

# The Psionic Method in Dental Medicine

The discussions so far have been concerned with the broad aspects of disease, but by no means an inconsiderable part of medical practice is concerned with dental hygiene in which psionic techniques afford normally unsuspected possibilities. There are two attitudes towards the problem of dental disorders, the preventative and the conservative, both of which are applied in their appropriate context.

The conditions of contemporary society inevitably throw the emphasis on the techniques of conservation. The dental surgeon is faced with immediate and pressing demands for the salvage of teeth which have already been attacked by disease, often irremediably; in the course of which new techniques of pain relief and mechanical restoration are evolved, with an expanding array of materials and equipment.

It would be fair to say, however, that the average practitioner regards salvage as the least satisfactory aspect of his skill and endeavours to apply his knowledge to prevention. There are two schools of thought here. One believes that dental disorders are largely the fault of the environment, so that although restorative surgery has a certain preventive value in ensuring adequate masticatory functioning (and aesthetic satisfaction) it must be reinforced by good oral hygiene, and proper stimulation of the dental supporting tissues.

In this category is the controversial subject of fluoridation of public water supplies. It has been claimed that the application of trace concentrations of fluorine preparations to the teeth prevents dental caries. Scientific evidence is divided concerning these claims and many regard them as non-proven or even potentially dangerous. The debate continues.

On a similar note, there is the vexing question of mercury amalgams. The body of research is steadily increasing which suggests that the use of mercury is outdated and positively dangerous for some people. It is the experience of many psionic practitioners that mercury toxicity can produce or contribute to many conditions affecting the central nervous system and distant parts of the body. Unfortunately, wholesale removal of old fillings and replacement with modern alternatives can sometimes be hazardous, because of the release of the toxins all at once. Indeed, there is evidence that when amalgam fillings need to be removed, there may be a correct order in which this should be done.

Apart from these issues, however, there is the aspect of diet and nutrition. The ecologists consider that here lies the key — or at least a major portion of it — to unlock the door to health and ensure prevention of disease, dental or otherwise. A great deal has been said and written on this subject, from the simple advice to avoid excesses, or to cut out refined carbohydrates and other processed and chemically contaminated foods, or to adopt a predominantly or total vegetarian diet.

It is argued, with justification, that the ways of life of contemporary society in industrialised communities are not likely to produce an environment in which a state of health can flourish. Even the physical activity necessary for healthy metabolic exchange is at a premium in a world in which mechanical transport and mechanical aids in general usurp almost all normal human functions.

In the face of these conditions one must surely look elsewhere for solutions. This is the view of the holistic school, which seeks a deeper understanding of the background to the distressingly prevalent troubles. Dental disorders are seen as merely specific and localised departures from overall health, so that the problem resolves itself into the location of the underlying causes of such departure, and the discovery of means whereby it may be prevented or at least ameliorated.

It is here that psionic methods are invaluable, and once again we can quote Carl Upton, whose training and subsequent experience as a salvage dentist did not satisfy his intuitive belief in the need to study the causes of the disorders, to which he found the key in the work of George Laurence.

### Carl Upton LDS (Birm), FIPsiMed (1910–1996)

Carl Upton did more than any other man to promote the pioneering work of Dr George Laurence. For many years he was the driving force behind both the Society and the Institute of Psionic Medicine.

Born into an English farming family, Carl Upton entered the Medical Faculty of Birmingham University where he studied dentistry in the Dental School of the Faculty. Throughout his training the emphasis was on the need for close collaboration with medical colleagues at all times, which materially influenced his outlook. After qualifying he spent two years in private practice before entering the Army Medical Service, in which he served for eight years at home and in the Middle East. He was then posted to the War Office as Deputy Assistant Director, Army Dental Service, which occupied him during the second half of the war.

At the close of the war he was sent for training in maxillo-facial dental surgery at the Victoria Hospital, East Grinstead, under Sir Archibald McIndoe, and was subsequently appointed Command Specialist Dental Surgeon to a home command, and later to India and Singapore. In 1948 he retired from the Army and entered private practice in South Africa, where he stayed for some years, working in close collaboration with his medical colleagues in local hospitals.

During this period he developed an increasing interest in the preventive aspects of dentistry, and took every opportunity to investigate any ideas, whether orthodox or not, that could throw light on the basic causes of dental disorders, in the pursuit of which he was greatly assisted by his wide travels and meetings with people of many cultures. On his return to England in 1963 he increasingly devoted his attention to the possibilities of homoeopathy in relation to dental conditions; and, having come into contact with Westlake, and later Laurence, he realised that the fulfilment of his quest lay in the integrated philosophy of Psionic Medicine.

Carl first met Laurence, who was then 86, in 1966. He soon proved to be his star pupil. Bringing with him many of his own insights into health and illness, he worked with Laurence to stream-line the whole diagnostic and treatment procedures into what is now known as the *Laurence-Upton technique* of psionic analysis.

In 1968 he retired from active dental practice to devote his attention to the furtherance of the reconciliation between medical science and the traditional healing arts, to which Psionic Medicine holds such an important key. In that year the Psionic Medical Society was formed.

Later, when Laurence asked him to develop a training pro-gramme for doctors and dentists, he initiated the formation of the Institute of Psionic Medicine with its power to grant Membership and Fellowship status to properly qualified candidates and to con-sider research projects.

Carl was the first secretary of both the Society and the Institute. He saw the need to document the proceedings of both bodies, and invited Dr Aubrey Westlake, whose book *The Pattern of Health* had inspired so many practitioners, to edit a Society journal. He was also the link man between a patient, who wished Dr Laurence's work to be recorded for the wider public, and J.H. Reyner, author, scientist and philosopher, whose book entitled *Psionic Medicine* (and in which he collaborated with both George Laurence and Carl Upton), was first published in 1974. The enlarged, updated second edition appeared in 1982 with additions, an appendix on bioplasm and associated clinical indications written by Carl. In addition, as a researcher (and as a later editor of the *Journal of the Psionic Medical Society and the Institute of Psionic Medicine*) he published many papers, articles and pamphlets, which have significantly added to the literature on the subject.

Several of the current psionic practitioners were fortunate enough to have been taught by Carl, who was able to provide a balancing picture of what is offered in both Eastern philosophy and Western science. The following paper originally published by the Psionic Medical Society gives his views of how Psionic Medicine may be used in dental practice.

Carl continued in active psionic medical practice until shortly before his death in 1996.

## The psionic method in preventive dental medicine

'Laurence, with his extensive knowledge of clinical morbid anatomy, physiology and pathology, combined with the experience derived from his researches into what he refers to as the "formative forces", has been able to establish definite causal relationships between disturbances produced in the formative body by certain diseases or infections, and clinical symptoms, usually of chronic disease, in the physical body.

'Under the influence of a scientific outlook devoted solely to a consideration of the structure of matter and its behaviour, medical and dental practice is conditioned to observe and treat the physicochemical organism within the limits of the technical knowledge in which it has been educated. Since knowledge of the vital dynamic forces involved in nature does not fall within these limits, medicine and dentistry have been deprived, other than in the case of a real intuitive clinical sense developed through long clinical experience, of the opportunity to come to grips with and understand the deep inherent causes of disease which lie in the vital being of man.

'Whereas observation of the physical personality can be carried out with the aid of the five senses and with the assistance of laboratory techniques and instruments, that of the vital force determining the nature of the individual can only be achieved through the use of a different range of senses, involving the exercise of the psionic faculty.

'Every doctor and dentist knows that the influences involved in heredity play a fundamental part in the make-up of their patient's constitution. They do not necessarily know the character of these influences. They are not thus aware of the nature of the unsuspected causes of ill-health that stem from the chain of inheritance; unless they have turned their attention in the direction indicated by Hahnemann and Laurence.

'To understand dental disease it is necessary to examine not only the relationship between the person and his environment and the character of that environment, but also to probe the relationship between the physical person and his vital essence. If this can be done then dental practice takes on a very different meaning — a new dimension is added.

'Although the immediate salvage necessity may remain, including modifications to the environment wherever desirable and possible, parallel with this, treatment can be instituted with a view to the correction of inherent causes, which are giving rise to a weakness in the structure, and to faulty metabolism of the dental tissues.

'Laurence has shown that not only the influences of serious disease in a forebear can disturb the balance of the *personal psi-field* of later generations, expressing as miasms, but that certain infectious diseases have their immediate effect in producing what he refers to as *'hangovers'* or Acquired Dynamic Toxins in the formative body. Both constitute causative factors, which must be eliminated before cure in the real sense of the word is possible. From the dental point of view, however meticulous the salvage operations or care in choice of food and way of life, the patient remains constantly at risk of dental lesions while miasms and dynamic toxins remain unresolved.

'Over an increasing number of cases diagnosed and treated by the psionic method where dental disorders occur, the high, almost universal, incidence of the tubercular miasms is noted. Although both human and bovine miasms are frequently present, there is evidence, not yet fully confirmed, that the miasms of bovine tuberculosis are especially significant as a possible predisposition to dental caries.

'Both the miasms and the acquired dynamic toxin associated with *measles* also occur very frequently. Less frequent are the miasms of *syphilis* and *gonorrhoea*. Among the acquired dynamic toxins regularly encountered are those associated with *staphylococcus aureus, streptococcus, E. coli, proteus, gaertner, morgan, bacillus catarrhalis, poliomyelitis* and the toxins related to *vaccination* and *aluminium*. It is not yet confirmed that all of these have any direct bearing on dental disorders, although without doubt the E. coli and vaccinosis toxins are significant in predisposing to paradontal conditions.

'It is considered of great importance, now we have the techniques of Psionic Medicine, that the diagnosis and elimination of miasms and acquired toxins in children should be carried out wherever possible and on an increasing scale as trained operators become available. Not only do children respond so readily and so effectively to this treatment but what is of far reaching benefit, the chain of miasms is broken. Children so treated are no longer "carriers" of inimical influences and thus ensure for their own children a better expectancy of health from the outset. During adolescence and child-bearing years any acquired dynamic toxins arising from acute infections or other causes should be eliminated. Deficiency of any of the active elements, vitamins or essential minerals, which often accompanies a disturbance in the psi-field, requires to be made good.

'It is evident from these remarks that psionic techniques provide valuable assistance in combating the modern scourge of debilitating dental disease. This arises from the introduction of a new dimension into the therapy, as may be illustrated clinically from practical experience in relation to dental caries.

'In the narrowest sense, the clinical picture presented by this disease is a breakdown in the hard dental tissues. Mechanical techniques are used to remove diseased tissues and provide substitute functional restorations. This is the main field in which the dental surgeon works, but the scope of his inquiry is widened by consideration of environmental factors. Poor local hygiene and dietetic imbalance are known to play a role in the production of tissue breakdown, so that in addition to mechanical restoration increasing attention is being given to preventive measures.

'Such measures, however, are still concerned with physical causation, whereas psionic techniques introduce a different dimension of diagnosis and treatment. In a large number of cases showing the incidence of dental caries psionic medical analysis has demonstrated the presence of inherited miasms. These are usually of the tubercular, particularly the bovine group, as already mentioned. In other words there is a genetic predisposition to the disease of dental caries. This of course may have been long suspected by dental clinicians but the nature and cause of the predisposition has not been apparent from work in the purely physical aspects of diagnosis and therapy. It has required the introduction of the new dimension opened up by psionic medical techniques to arrive at an understanding of basic factors involved in the causation of the disease and the means of its eradication.

'Whereas dental surgical techniques and environmental preventive measures have succeeded in raising the level of dental functional efficiency to a certain point they have not been able to reduce the incidence of the disease from the genetic standpoint. This now becomes possible through psionic diagnosis and the removal of the causative miasms concerned.

'For the dental surgeon who wishes to add this new dimension to his practice, the basic necessities are a knowledge of the homoeopathic *Materia Medica* and an ability to employ the psionic faculty, both of which require a period of training. But with such equipment the treatment can be of a far more comprehensive and deeper nature, taking into account the whole man, with which one is fundamentally concerned in the pursuit of health.'

# 14

# Psionic Veterinary Medicine

Mark Elliott BVSc, VetMFHom, MRCVS, MIPsiMed

*'If the physician clearly perceives what is to be cured in disease...if he clearly perceives what is curative in medicines...and if he knows how to adapt, according to clearly defined principles, what is curative in medicines to what he has discovered to be undoubtedly morbid in the patient, so that recovery must ensue...if finally, he knows the obstacles to recovery in each case and is aware how to remove them, so that the restoration may be permanent: then he understands how to treat judiciously and rationally, and he is a true practitioner of the healing art.'*

**Hahnemann, Organon of Medicine fifth edition (1893)**

This statement by Samuel Hahnemann summarises the aims of all true Homoeopaths and is adhered to with zeal by many. However, the common stumbling block in any practice is in perceiving what is to be cured and how to remove the obstacles to recovery. Nowhere is this truer than in the world of veterinary medicine, where the patients can rarely communicate directly with the practitioner. Hahnemann, in later life, found that a good number of chronic disease patterns failed to cure according to the basic doctrines of homoeopathy, and that the diseases increased from year to year in their hold on the patient, and hence in their severity. Hahnemann found that there were three main *patterns* to these chronic diseases, and called them Syphilis, Sycosis and Psora. Whilst these three miasmatic trends, or a combination of them, can be identified to some extent in human patients, it is extremely difficult to do so in animals and, without removal of these blockages to cure, one cannot ever achieve the success one would like in treating animal patients. Psionic Medicine offers a real and positive approach to identifying and tackling these problems in animal patients.

In more recent times there have been other 'miasms' identified giving rise to theories that there are many more patterns of blockage to the curative forces within the body. However, if one analyses these, I believe one always comes back to Hahnemann's basic three disease *patterns*, and that the 'new' miasms are really combinations of the three main trends, in varying proportions of significance, coloured in their effects by the imposition of external influences on the body from modern life. Nowhere is the effect of modern living more obvious than in our pets today. The average cat or dog suffers constant unnecessary vaccination, whilst fed on a diet of reconstituted waste product 'preserved' with carcinogenic and health-debilitating chemicals. The amount of sickness seen in domestic animals is staggering as a result. Just putting a dog on a natural diet of raw meat and vegetables in appropriate amounts will improve or cure 40 percent of disease in my experience. Worryingly this can only mirror the future for Man as he is slowly educated by the media to consume more and more processed, chemically preserved and genetically modified food.

As these 'new' miasms can be considered in animals to be patterns, rather than the specific diseases of Hahnemann's day, the witnesses used in human psionic medical dowsing have great validity in identifying disease trends and patterns and hence ways to treat a patient. This brings us full circle back to McDonagh's theories suggesting that each is a pattern of the expansion, or contraction, of protein which leads to energetic imbalance and hence disease. Only once these imbalances are corrected will health occur, or will one be able to give a homoeopathic remedy, constitutionally prescribed, to assist the beleaguered body back to a healthy state.

To understand this argument it is best to first consider the miasms separately, and to superimpose psionic findings from practice and real-life patients onto the concepts.

## The Syphilitic miasm

Syphilitic type diseases are characterised by a chronic, desperate struggle where the body is destroying itself in an attempt to survive. Classically *ulceration* and *collapse of structure* is seen, as the disease is not manageable. Psychosis, aggression, and anti-social behaviour all are identifiable with this miasm.

Often these patterns are seen in later life.

*Tissues affected*: Glands, Bone and CNS. The embryological derivation of these tissues is Ectodermal and congenital agenesis can be a sign.

*Mental states include*: Delusions, suspicion, aggression, fear of attack.

*Common physical symptoms include*: those with aggravations at night, for storms and for cold and heat. Improvements are made when the patient is moving and when cold is applied. Poor healing of wounds, offensive smells to skin complaints and weak joints are also common. Neonatal opthalmia in puppies is a symptom of the problem, deriving from the parents, and nowhere is this more obvious than in the Welsh Springer Spaniel where this is common along with epilepsy, neuroses, poor/no formation of adequate hips, and where direct lines of inheritance are easily shown.

*Modern veterinary equivalents include*: Bovine Spongiform Encephalopathy, Ovine Scrapie, Feline Aids, Canine Parvovirus and its vaccine, Feline Enteritis (a parvovirus) and its vaccine, Canine Distemper virus and its vaccine, Equine Herpes virus and its vaccine, many autoimmune diseases, nerve degeneration, lymphatic disease, Equine foal epiphysitis.

It is interesting to note that the work of Susan Wynn DVM (unpublished to date) on Canine Distemper and Parvovirus vaccine has shown a direct tendency to destroy the thyroid gland in some breed lines — proof of the destructive nature of vaccines and of this miasm — and this work has directly been linked with that of Jean Dodds DVM showing the tendency of canine vaccines to cause autoimmune disease (Dodds, W.J. 1983).

*Commonly assumed remedies* by classical homoeopaths include Mercury, Acid nit, Aurum and the Heavy Metals, Kali bich, Asafoetida, Phytolacca.

## The Sycotic miasm

Sycotic diseases show as a hyper-response arising out of a *deficiency* of the normal immune system response e.g., Tumours and other proliferative diseases, and some allergies. That is, there is an over-response by the body inadequately controlled by normal mechanisms. Neurosis.

Often these patterns are seen in the middle of life.

*Tissues affected*: Liver, Pancreas, Thyroid, Parathyroid and thymic parenchyma. Linings of the GI Tract, Eustachian tube and middle ear, respiratory system, urinary system and glands derived from it e.g. Prostate.

The embryological derivation of these tissues is generally meso-dermal or endodermal.

*Mental states include*: Despair, indifference, antisocial behaviour, fixed habits and obsessions, jealousy, cruelty.

*Common physical symptoms include*: Warts, tumours, affections of the mucous membranes, poor digestive function, symptoms worse for cold and animals which fail to thrive, inflammations of the reproductive organs, eye affections, sterility, inflammatory joint disease with wandering pains worse for damp, exfoliative skin disease, psoriasis, some asthma especially with loss of smell, muco-purulent discharges.

*Modern veterinary equivalents include*: Feline Leukaemia virus and its vaccine. Rabies vaccine (now the cause of many canine skin tumours in the USA). Much skin disease seen in dogs. Feline Miliary Eczema (although the work of Elliott, 1992, suggests this may be an iatrogenically sparked recrudescence of a dormant miasm), Ringworm, testicular tumours and many of the behavioural problems seen in practice. (On a cynical note here the syphilitic miasm-associated aggression often leads to euthanasia so less are seen for therapy.) Canine transmissible venereal tumours. Equine Sarcoids, interdigital dermatitis in cattle and sheep, and Feline Hyperthyroidism.

*Commonly assumed remedies* by classical homoeopaths include Thuja, Natrum sulph, Cinnabaris, Sepia, Kali sulph, Acid nit, Staphysagria, Lycopodium, and to these I would add Pulsatilla in animals which has both Anti-Sycotic and Anti-Syphilitic tendencies, and also Arsenicum alb for its feeling of vulnerability and its well-known aggravations.

A favourite summary of mine for this miasm is *perverted functional activity*.

## The Psoric miasm

Psoric diseases are characterised by a constant, inadequate struggle to heal, a deficiency in the response of the vital force. Classically the reaction of the body is manifest in those parts of the body dealing with the outside world — Skin, Nervous system, and Gut. *Functional disturbances. Deficiency Disease.*

Often these types of disease are seen in the earlier part of life, before the vital force gives up its unequal struggle and tends to one of the other miasma. At this stage the process is not life-threatening, or hopeless (unless tackled by the modern medical approach with steroids, piling suppressive medication on hypo-function, and driving disease deeper internally and miasmatically).

*Tissues affected*: Skin, Intestine and other Mucous membranes. Nervous system. The embryological derivation of these tissues is mostly ectoderm.

*Mental states include*: Anticipatory anxiety, fearfulness.

*Common physical symptoms include*: Dry, persistent eczema, weakness of function and of tissues, chilliness, dirtiness with a dread of bathing (but not with the foul discharges of Sycosis), increased compensatory appetite, poor healing and tendency to easy injury. Enlarged lymph nodes.

*Modern veterinary equivalents include*: Atopy and other allergic skin and Intestinal diseases, Mange, Meningitis, illness after a loss and recurrent infections of unknown origin suggest this miasm. COPD (Broken wind) in horses.

Many of the remedies commonly used classically are inorganic compounds of trace elements, such as Calc carb, the Kali, Natrum, and Magnesium salts, Phosphorous, Silica, the Carbons, Arsenicum alb, Barium, and Cuprum, although some plant remedies are used such as Lycopodium and Mezereum as well as Psorinum the nosode itself. It is here the work of Jan Scholten on the elemental remedies comes into its own in the therapy of disease and I would state this is essential reading for anyone contemplating treating an animal homoeopathically.

Sankaran introduces the interesting aspect of linking the three chronic miasms to stages in our lives. He includes the acute miasm, which is youth. Responses are quick and illness can be easily thrown off...the threats are external with a strong instinctive reaction. During early adulthood there is still much energy, liveliness and activity (Psora), and the openness to express fear and anxiety. Situations are difficult; there is a struggle to succeed. There is hope and failure does not mean the end of the world. Then middle age sets in (Sycosis). We realise our limitations and to preserve face we start to cover up, hide our incapacities, to be accepted. Our reactions and habits are more fixed. This is something very true for our society. Wisdom and age are no longer valued. We are seen as resources and have a place as long as we keep up with the set pace. Once we start to crumble we are no longer valued so we try to hide this for as long as possible. Then comes old age (Syphilis), the time for letting go and decay. This is reflected in the syphilitic miasm. There is despair about recovery but, unlike Psora, without hope. Whilst this is difficult to anthropomorphise into veterinary medicine, the principles often seem to apply to the tendencies towards disease with age.

From these summarised descriptions of the three miasms, one can look at all chronic diseases (and I categorise all diseases which are not thrown off in five days as chronic), analyse their respective patterns and fit them into one or more of the types. Add into this the named diseases found to respond to appropriate therapies relating to the miasms and one is a long way to building the concepts of psionic medicine into modern veterinary medicine.

## Bioplasmic associations

In the human version of Psionic Medicine, many of the bioplasmic associations (best thought of as chronic recognisable tendencies following infectious disease, which may have happened in this life, or in a previous generation) are often now thought of as miasms in their own right. I prefer to think of them as sparks igniting one or more of the three main miasma (or disease patterns) to manifest in differing degrees as the body can only respond in the three fashions described by Hahnemann. However, the Hahnemannian principles of similia similibus curentor still apply and it is quite logical that either nosodes, or remedies producing similar patterns of disease, can be utilised to push the vital force in the right direction and achieve a cure. The psionic method of looking at historical causative factors is therefore like a traveller's guide to unravelling the complexities of the presenting aberrations of the vital force. One must accept that this is only one-way, but one logical to the medically trained mind. If one of the main three is discovered this obviously indicates that a major insult to the vital force has either been due to that disease, or its species-equivalent similars, and has firmly pushed the body towards that disease tendency, colouring the prescriber's decisions.

These associations are usually reflected in the findings on DNA and RNA when using the Laurence-Upton technique of analysis.

## Bioplasmic associations and their relevance in animals

*Tubercular miasm or toxin*: Found in all species, but more commonly cats and dogs. Symptoms include Asthma, Skin diseases, diabetes and problems in puppies with temper. Tub Koch has been a cause of a large stables suffering from back problems and respiratory dysfunction in a high percentage of the horses. This responded well to the nosode inside a week.

*Syphilitic miasm or toxin*: Found in all species (see Chap. 6 for more detail). The *only* finding yet in foals with epiphysitis. This is commonly thought to be a nutritional disease but all cases treated with Lueticum have so far responded within a few days. No direct syphilitic organism known.

*Gonorrhoea toxin*: The least commonly found of the main three miasms in animals and there is no equivalent disease. Not yet found in a horse or ruminant by myself. (see Chap. 6 for more detail).

*Measles toxin*: This is the equivalent of Canine Distemper and is a major miasm in this species as, for no logical reason, it is given as a vaccine annually by many vets. Symptoms include cardio-vascular disturbances (Cavalier King Charles Spaniels), Skin disorders, Hepatopathies, Chorea, Epilepsy, Senility and Hypo-thyroidism. Recently a case of a Harris Hawk showed this as a major factor and hence was prescribed for accordingly. It is known there are analogous viruses affecting birds.

*Staphylococcus*: A common toxin in all species causing respiratory and GI Tract symptoms poorly responsive to antibiotics. Often associated with skin disorders, its effects are felt throughout the body.

*Streptococcus*: It seems hardly an analysis goes by without this appearing. I have to question its significance in animals as I rarely treat it, unless cases are failing to improve, and it disappears often anyway once other miasmatic causes are treated. Significant only if cardio-vascular, neurological or musculo-skeletal symptoms exist.

*Bowel nosodes*: Of major importance in Canine and Equine patients who are nowadays fed on novel food types, rarely to their benefit. Of significance in almost all cases. For symptoms and associated remedies see the work of *Paterson* and the *Bowel Nosodes*. I would add somewhat to this work by adding the remedies Thuja, Anacardium and Sulphur to those for the treatment of Faecalis organisms in animals. I would offer these guidelines for prescribing: if the animal is quite ill and the main cause found psionically is a bowel nosode, give a high potency; if the animal is well give a longer course in low potency to clear the miasm, sometimes up to a month is required; if of some, but not major, significance give a 200c.

*Malaria*: Not found in the UK but may be of significance elsewhere.

*Klebsiella*: Found commonly as a miasm in affections of the articulations of the spine in dogs, and once by me in a horse.

*Aluminium*: Occasionally found as a problem in dogs and cats with the typical associated skin and gastric dysfunctions and wasting diseases.

*Vaccination*: A major problem in all species (see Chap. 6 to the main three miasm write-ups for more detail). In the USA (and now some areas of the UK) Leukaemia vaccine is now often injected into cats' legs rather than the neck as one can, apparently, amputate a leg once cancer sets in!

*Kennel Cough*: A multifactorial disease, which often leads to chronic bronchitic and pleuritic states if treated with the usual antibiotics and steroids. This can seem to have some generational hangover.

*Herpes*: Found psionically as a problem only in cats and horses. In the former it tends to nasal and respiratory disease, while in the latter musculo-skeletal problems, fertility and respiratory problems are all associated.

*Viroids*: BSE, Scrapie, Feline BSE, etc., all arise from time to time, and are treated generally with nosodes or as syphilitic miasms.

In all animals chemical preservatives and colourants in food are significant causes of disease, acting at all levels. Many of the additives are banned in the human food chain for their side effects and carcinogenic properties. It is worth looking for these in an analysis and also for the mineral and tissue depletions often arising out of being fed the same processed diet day in, day out. In addition animals are extremely sensitive to *geopathic stress* and persistent cases should always have this considered. Emotional distress is very significant, it is interesting to note that most rescued dogs itch and this is often a Psora manifesting, with an appropriate mineral solution.

## The psionic analysis

The technique of analysis is taught from one practitioner to another and so not detailed here. It is sufficient to say that the original technique is as appropriate for animals as it is for humans, although the witness cards vary somewhat to reflect the bioplasmic associations relevant.

## In summary

The use of psionic analytical techniques is highly relevant in today's rapid and stressful world. Animals and their owners are under increasing environmental, chemical, and disease pressure and one can only hope to achieve high levels of success in patients that cannot talk if one can perceive what one needs to treat in the patient. Without it I couldn't have built my practice, nor developed a real understanding of what Homoeopathy is capable of achieving.

This work is but a start at collating the vast amount of data that the use of Psionic Medicine will, I hope, reveal for animals.

## Reference
Flint G. *Yorkshire Medicine*, (1991) Winter edn.
Hahnemann S. *Organon of Medicine*, (1893) 5th edn.
Dodds W.J. Vaccine safety and efficacy revisited. *Veterinary Forum*, (1983) May 68–71
Elliott M. *Homoeopathic treatment of Feline Miliary Eczema*. (1992) BAHVS Conference.

## Further reading
1. J.H. Reyner *Psionic Medicine*, First edition 1974, second edition 1982
2. Aubrey Westlake *The Pattern of Health*, 1961
3. David Tansley D.C. *Radionics, Interface with the Ether Fields*, C.W. Daniel, 1981
4. George Laurence FRSC, The Unitary Conception of Disease in Relation to Radiesthetic Diagnosis, 1967
5. Herbert A. Roberts *Principles and Art of Cure by Homoeopathy*, Health Science Press
6. Samuel Hahnemann *The Chronic Diseases Vols 1 and 2*, 1978
7. Sue Asquith and Elwyn Rees *Models, Methods, Mechanisms in Millennium Medicine*, 1998
8. R. Sankaran *The Spirit of Homoeopathy*, 1981
9. J. Scholten *Homoeopathy and the Elements*, 1993
10. J. Paterson*The Bowel Nosodes*, 1950

'*Science without religion is lame, religion
without science is blind.*'

**Science, Philosophy and Religion: a Symposium 1941**
**Albert Einstein**

When I was a medical student many of the textbooks we used bore the names of illustrious members of the profession, many of whom had either long since retired from practice or had departed this life. Yet so important was their contribution to their chosen field that their names had seemingly become indelibly printed on the spines of the book. I often wondered just how much of their original writings were left in the new editions.

The original edition of *Psionic Medicine*, by J.H. Reyner, in collaboration with George Laurence and Carl Upton, appeared in 1974. An enlarged second edition was published in 1982, with updates by Carl Upton. Unfortunately, it has been out of print for some years. This fact prompted the Institute of Psionic Medicine to consider the production of a new book. There were a number of options available. To publish the book as it stood was dismissed, because there have been many changes in thinking since the last edition. To produce a completely new and different book was a possibility, yet it was felt that this would inevitably have to draw heavily on the original as a source. This effectively made up our minds for us: the new book should and would be an updated version of the last.

I now have much sympathy with the editors of those textbooks I pored over as a student. Trying to retain the original structure of a book yet fit new ideas into its matrix is no easy task. Yet it has, I feel, been the right thing to do. Keeping the original structure, at times reproducing papers and quotes from the original authorship, has permitted us to retain the historical documentation of the beginnings of Psionic Medicine. And it is instructive to hear George Laurence and Carl Upton unfurl their views and describe their cases.

Undoubtedly, the major addition to this book has been the chapter on the Psi-Field Hypothesis by Professor Ervin Laszlo. His concept and description of an all-encompassing, interconnecting field is a masterful synthesis of science, philosophy and wisdom. It is one of the most lucid and brilliant pieces of thinking, providing possible explanations to so many previously imponderable questions in science, philosophy and spirituality. It is *the* Grand Unified Theory.

There have, of course, been other great thinkers whose insights into Nature were inspired according to their time. Akenaten, Swedenborg, Hahnemann, Steiner, McDonagh and Jung were such men, and our consideration of them in this book illustrates how compatible their ideas were with Laszlo's Psi-Field Hypothesis.

The use of ancient Egyptian symbolism, in particular the pyramid and Akenaten's concept of the Aten, the sun-disk, must not be misconstrued as implying that Psionic Medicine is in any sense a spiritual or philosophical system. It is not; indeed it is no more spiritual or philosophical than western medicine or western surgery; the models are merely chosen because they serve to illustrate an idea.

But one of the beauties of the Psi-Field Hypothesis is the amount of ground which it covers. It is in no sense a spiritual concept. It offers no suggestion about deity or divinity, yet at the same time it is compatible with virtually any religion or philosophy. And, at the same time, it is compatible with the cutting edge of theoretical physics, the new biology, the most recent research in consciousness psychology, and parapsychology.

We as psionic practitioners welcome Laszlo's hypothesis, since it explains in scientific terms much about the nature of the pioneering approach developed by Dr George Laurence. The nature of non-locality, interconnectedness and the interaction between energy and matter, these are fundamental to Psionic Medicine. The personal psi-field becomes an obvious reality, just as tuning into the psi-field itself seems such a logical thing to do in order to help an individual to regain health.

It is a source of debate as to whether Psionic Medicine is a science or an art. There are some who would suggest that the use of a pendulum cannot be regarded as being in any way scientific. The thing is, however, that the pendulum is merely used as an indicator, an amplifier of an ideomotor response, which occurs when the operator uses one of his, or her, higher faculties to become active. The manner in which that indicator is used in an analytical fashion with quantifiable charts, specimens and witnesses, is absolutely scientific. The other side of the coin, of course, is the fact that one does have to develop a degree of adeptness. It is indeed a skill. On this basis, Psionic Medicine can perhaps best be described as a scientific art.

The Institute is aware of the need to perform research, and to validate, verify and publish its findings. The *Journal of the Psionic Medical Society and the Institute of Psionic Medicine* has always been used for publishing individual research, but an additional peer-reviewed journal is currently in preparation to document this part of our work. At the same time, Mr John Fryer, the secretary of the Psionic Medical Society, is transferring our archives onto disk, so that the entire literature appertaining to Psionic Medicine will become available to researchers.

The position regarding training was referred to in Chapter Nine. At this time such training is only available to doctors, dentists and veterinary surgeons with a registerable qualification in the UK.

It is important to reiterate that Psionic Medicine is not a panacea. It is a highly efficient, scientific means of finding the underlying causes of illness. If an illness has reached a point where structural change has taken place, with alteration or destruction of tissue, then it may not be possible to produce reversal of such pathology. However, by discovering the underlying cause of the illness and removing it homoeopathically (or whichever way is indicated) at the very least the ongoing 'process' which is causing the pathology and the structural change may be halted. The body's natural homoeostatic or self-healing mechanisms may then do the best that they can.

One thing is certain: this book will not be the final word. We as psionic practitioners will continue to search and research. Our motto is apt — *Tolle Causam* — Seek the Cause.

# Selected Bibliography

The following works have been used as references in each of the chapters, or are books which will give the interested reader further information about the topics covered.

## Chapter One

Bohm, David, *Wholeness and the Implicate Order*, Routledge & Kegan Paul, London, 1980

Capra, Fritjof, *The Tao of Physics (Third Edition)*, Shambhala, Boston, 1991

Capra, Fritjof, *The Web of Life*, Harper Collins, London, 1997

Chopra, Deepak, *Quantum Healing — Exploring the Frontiers of Mind/Body Medicine*, Bantam Books, New York, 1990

Gerber, Richard, *Vibrational Medicine*, Bear & Co, Santa Fe, 1988

Hancock, Graham and Faiia, Santha, *Heaven's Mirror-Quest for the Lost Civilization*, Michael Joseph, London, 1998

Laszlo, Ervin, *The Whispering Pond*, Element, Shaftesbury, Dorset, 1996

Laszlo, Ervin, *The Creative Cosmos*, Floris Books, Edinburgh, 1994

Lovelock, James, *Gaia — A New Look at Life on Earth*, Oxford University Press, Oxford, 1979

Pert, Candace, *Molecules of Emotion*, Pocket Books, London, 1997

Sheldrake, Rupert, *New Science of Life*, Blond & Briggs, London, 1981

Watkins, Alan, *Mind-Body Medicine — a Clinician's Guide to Psychoneuroimmunology*, Churchill Livingstone, London, 1997

## Chapter Two

Grof, Stanislav, *The Adventure of Self-Discovery*, Albany: The State University of New York Press, 1988.

Laszlo, Ervin, *The Creative Cosmos*, Edinburgh, Floris Books, 1993

Laszlo, Ervin, *The Interconnected Universe*, Singapore and London: World Scientific, 1995

Laszlo, Ervin, *The Whispering Pond*, Rockport, Shaftesbury and Brisbane, 1996


## Chapter Three

Bronowsky, Jacob, *The Ascent of Man*, BBC, London, 1973

Jones, Ernest, *The Life and Work of Sigmund Freud*, Pelican, London, 1961

Lyons, Albert and Petrucelli, Joseph, *Medicine — an Iillustrated History*, Abradale Press, New York, 1987

Pert, Candace, *Molecules of Emotion*, Pocket Books, London, 1997

Poynter Noël, *Medicine and Man*, Pelican, London, 1971

Rhodes, Philip, *An Outline History of Medicine*, Butterworths, London, 1985

Souter, Keith, *Cure Craft — Traditional Folk Remedies and Treatment from Antiquity to the Present Day*, C.W. Daniel, Saffron Walden, Essex, 1995

Walker, Kenneth, *Patients and Doctors*, Pelican, London, 1957


## Chapter Four

Burr, Harold Saxton, *Blueprint for Immortality — the Electric Patterns of Life*, C.W. Daniel, Saffron Walden, Essex, 1972

Collinge, William, *Subtle Energy*, Thorsons, London, 1998

Frazer, Sir James, *The Golden Bough*, Wordsworth, Ware, Hertfordshire, 1993

Gerber, Richard, *Vibrational Medicine*, Bear & Co, Santa Fe, 1988

Osho, *In Search of the Miraculous — Chakras, Kundalini and the Seven Bodies*, C.W. Daniel, Saffron Walden, Essex, 1996

Ozaniec, Naomi, *The Elements of the Chakras*, Element, Shaftesbury, Dorset, 1997

Steiner, Rudolph, *Theosophy — an Introduction...*, Rudolph Steiner Press, London 1970

Steiner, Rudolph, *The Philosophy of Freedom*, Rudolph Steiner Press, London, 1979

Tansley. David, *Radionics and the Subtle Anatomy of Man*, C.W. Daniel, Saffron Walden, Essex, 1972

Tansley, David, *Radionics: Science or Magic?* C.W. Daniel, Saffron Walden, Essex, 1982

Tansley, David, *Ray Paths and Chakra Gateways*, C.W. Daniel, Saffron Walden, Essex, 1985

Tansley, David, *Chakras — Rays and Radionics*, C.W.Daniel, Essex, 1988

## Chapter Five

Bach, Edward, *The Twelve Healers and Other Remedies*, C.W. Daniel, Saffron Walden, Essex, 1983

Bach, Edward, *Heal Thyself*, C.W. Daniel, Saffron Walden, Essex, 1984

Campbell, Anthony, *The Two faces of Homoeopathy*, Jill Norman, London, 1984

Close, Stuart, *The Genius of Homoeopathy — Lectures and Essays on Homoeopathic Philosophy*, B. Jain, Delhi, India, 1996

Hahnemann, Samuel, *Organon of Medicine*, 5th and 6th edns, B. Jain, Delhi, India, 1994

Hobhouse, Rosa, *Life of Christian Samuel Hahnemann*, B. Jain, Delhi, India, 1995

Kent, James Tyler, *Lectures on Homoeopathic Materia Medica*, Homoeopathic Publications, New Delhi, 1980

Modi, Sanjay, *Organon of Medicine Simplified (Degree course syllabus)*, B. Jain, Delhi, India, 1989

Souter, Keith, *Homoeopathy for the Third Age — Treatment for People in Middle and Later Life*, C.W. Daniel, Saffron Walden, Essex, 1993

Souter, Keith, *Homoeopathy; Heart and Soul — Treatment for Emotional Problems*, C.W. Daniel, Saffron Walden, Essex, 1995

Souter, Keith, *The Art of Homoeopathy*, B. Jain, Delhi, India, 1996

Vithoulkas, George, *Homoeopathy — Medicine of the New Man*, Thorsons, Wellingborough, 1979

Weeks, Nora, *The Medical Discoveries of Edward Bach, Physician*, C.W. Daniel, Saffron Walden, Essex, 1973

## Chapter Six

Bailey, A., Treatise on the Seven Rays, 1925

Burnett, J.C., *A New Cure of Consumption*, 1906

Hahnemann, S.C,. *The Chronic Diseases*, 1828

Kent, J.T., *Lectures on Homoeopathic Philosophy* No. 19 (reprint) 1976

Paterson, J., *The Bowel Nosodes*, 1950

Sankaran, R., *The Spirit of Homoeopathy*, 1982

Shepherd, D., *A Physician's Posy*, C.W. Daniel, 1969

Westlake, A, A New Dimension in Medicine, *Psionic Medicine* Nos 11 & 12, 1976 & 1977

## Chapter Seven

McDonagh, J.R. *Protein — the Basis of all Life*, Heinemann, London, 1966

Reyner, J.H., Laurence, George and Upton, Carl, *Psionic Medicine — the Study and Treatment of the Causative Factors in Illness*, 2nd edn, Routledge & Kegan Paul, London, 1982

## Chapter Eight

Bolton, Brett, *Edgar Cayce Speaks*, Avon, New York, 1969

Fenwick, Peter and Fenwick, Elizabeth, *Past Lives — an Investigation Into Reincarnation Memories*, Headline, London, 1999

Griffon, T. Wynne, *History of the Occult*, Grange, London, 1991

Guiley, Rosemary, *Encyclopedia of Mystical & Paranormal Experience*, Grange, London, 1991

Hitching, Francis, *Dowsing — the Psi Connection*, Doubleday, New York, 1978

Lorimer, David, *Whole in One: The Near-Death Experience and the Ethic of Interconnectedness*, Arkana, London, 1990

Miller, George, *Psychology — the Science of Mental Life*, Penguin, 1972

Osho, *And Now, and Here — on Death, Dying and Past Lives*, C.W. Daniel, Saffron Walden, Essex, 1995

Reyner, J.H., Laurence, George and Upton, Carl, *Psionic Medicine — the Study and Treatment of the Causative Factors in Illness*, 2nd edn, Routledge & Kegan Paul, London, 1982

Rolfe, Mona, *The Spiral of Life — Cycles of Reincarnation*, C.W. Daniel, Saffron Walden, Essex, 1981

Rolfe, Mona, *Initiation by the Nile*, C.W. Daniel, Saffron Walden, Essex, 1986

## Chapter Nine

Copen, Bruce and Kowa, Willi, *The Pendulum*, Academic Publications, Haywards Heath, Sussex, 1986

Hitching, Francis, *Dowsing — the Psi Connection*, Doubleday, New York, 1978

Nielsen, Greg and Polansky, Joseph, *Pendulum Power*, Aquarian, Wellingborough, Northamptonshire, 1986

Reyner, J.H., Laurence, George and Upton, Carl, *Psionic Medicine — the Study and Treatment of the Causative Factors in Illness*, 2nd edn, Routledge & Kegan Paul, London, 1982

Tansley, David V. *Radionics and the Subtle Anatomy of Man*, C.W. Daniel, Saffron Walden, Essex, 1972

## Chapter Ten

Bach, Edward, *The Twelve Healers and Other Remedies*, C.W. Daniel, Saffron Walden, Essex, 1983

Bailey, Arthur, *Dowsing for Health — the Applications & Methods for Holistic Healing*, Quantum, London, 1990

Copen, Bruce and Kowa, Willi, *The Pendulum*, Academic Publications, Haywards Heath, Sussex, 1986

Chandu, Jack, *The Pendulum Book*, C.W. Daniel, Saffron Walden, Essex, 1988

Hitching, Francis, *Dowsing — the Psi Connection*, Doubleday, New York, 1978

Howard, Judy, *The Bach Flower Remedies Step by Step*, C.W. Daniel, Saffron Walden, Essex, 1993

Nielsen, Greg and Polansky, Joseph, *Pendulum Power*, Aquarian, Wellingborough, Northamptonshire, 1986

Reyner, J.H., Laurence, George and Upton, Carl, *Psionic Medicine — the Study and Treatment of the Causative Factors in Illness*, 2nd edn, Routledge & Kegan Paul, London, 1982

Spiesberger, Karl, *Reveal the Power of the Pendulum*, Foulsham, London, 1987

Wethered, Vernon, *An Introduction to Medical Radiesthesia & Radionics*, C.W. Daniel, Saffron Walden, Essex, 1987

Wethered, Vernon, *The Practice of Medical Radiesthesia*, C.W. Daniel, Saffron Walden, Essex, 1987

## Chapter Eleven

Gilbert, Peter, *A Doctor's Guide to Helping Yourself with Biochemic Tissue Salts*, Thorsons, Wellingborough, Northamptonshire, 1984

Reyner, J.H., Laurence, George., Upton, Carl, *Psionic Medicine — the Study and Treatment of the Causative Factors in Illness*, 2nd edn, Routledge & Kegan Paul, London, 1982

Stanway, Andrew, *A Guide to Biochemic Tissue Salts*, Van Dyke Books, Redhill, Surrey, 1982

# *Further Reading*
# *From Second Edition*

Bradbury, Parnell, *Adventures in Healing*, Neville Spearman, London, 1969

Broderick, F.W., *Dental Medicine*, Kimpton, London, 1939

Burnet, Sir Macfarlane, *Genes, Dreams and Realities*, Medical & Technical Publishing Company, London, 1971

Carrel, Alexis, *Man, the Unknown*, Hamish Hamilton, London, 1935

Hauschka, Rudolph, *The Nature of Substance*, trans: Mary Richards and Marjorie Spock, Vincent Stuart, London, 1966

Heywood, R., *Beyond the Reach of Sense*, Dutton, New York, 1961

Koestler, A., *The Roots of Coincidence*, Hutchinson, London, 1972

McDonagh, J.R., *Protein — The Basis of All Life*, Heinemann, London, 1966

Mermet, The Abbé Alexis, *Principles and Practice of Radiesthesia*, trans: Mark Clement, Vincent Stuart, London, 1959

Pachter, Henry, *Paracelsus*, Henry Schuman, New York, 1951

Rawson, D.S., 'A Homoeopathic Approach to Pollution', *Journal of the American Institute of Homoeopathy*, 1972, 65 (2)

Reyner, J.H., *No Easy Immortality*, George Allen & Unwin, London, 1979

Rhine, L.E., *Hidden Channels of the Mind*, Sloane, New York, 1961

Richards, Guyon, *The Chain of Life*, Health Science Press, London, 1973

Roberts, H.A., *The Principles and Art of Cure by Homoeopathy*, Health Science Press, London, 1972

Schwaller, R.A., *Symbol and the Symbolic*, Autumn Press, Massachusetts, 1978

Sherrington, Sir Charles, *Man on his Nature*, Cambridge University Press, London, 1940. A wide-ranging expression of a biologist's philosophy originally given as the Gifford Lectures to the University of Edinburgh in 1937–8. Reprinted in Pelican Edition.

Tomlinson, H., *The Divination of Disease*, Health Science Press, London, 1953

Watson, Lyall, *Supernature*, Hodder, London, 1973

Westlake, A.T., *The Pattern of Health*, Revised Edition, 1973, Shambhala, San Francisco, 1961. Personal experiences with paranormal phenomena, including an account of the secret science of the Kahunas of Polynesia.

Westlake, A.T., *Life threatened — Menace and Way Out*, Stuart & Watkins, London, 1971

Wheeler, Charles and Kenyon, J.D., *Introduction to the Principles and Practice of Homoeopathy*, Health Science Press, London, 1972

# Useful Addresses

**The Psionic Medical Society**
The Society exists to support research into the causes of chronic and 'incurable' disease, its prevention, and the advancement of, and training in, methods of diagnosis and treatment, including the homoeopathic, which are known to be free of toxic risk.

Mr John Fryer,
52 Honeysuckle Close,
Badger Farm,
Winchester,
Hants, SO22 4QQ

**The Institute of Psionic Medicine**
Training in the techniques of Psionic Medicine is available to Medical, Dental and Veterinary practitioners.

For a list of qualified practitioners or information about training contact:

Dr Pam Tatham,
79 Hallgarth Street,
Durham, DH1 3AY

**The British Society of Dowsers**
Sycamore Barn,
Hastingleigh,
Ashford,
Kent, TN25 5HW

# Index